T0134536

Practical Anesthetic Management

C. Philip Larson Jr. • Richard A. Jaffe

Practical Anesthetic Management

The Art of Anesthesiology

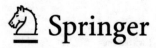

C. Philip Larson Jr., MDCM
Professor Emeritus, Anesthesia and
    Neurosurgery Stanford University
Professor of Clinical Anesthesiology (Ret.)
David Geffen School of Medicine at UCLA
Los Angeles, CA, USA

Richard A. Jaffe, MD, PhD
Professor of Anesthesiology
    and Neurosurgery
Stanford University School of Medicine
Stanford, CA, USA

Videos can also be accessed at http://link.springer.com/book/10.1007/978-3-319-42866-6.

ISBN 978-3-319-82684-4   ISBN 978-3-319-42866-6   (eBook)
DOI 10.1007/978-3-319-42866-6

© Springer International Publishing Switzerland 2017
Softcover reprint of the hardcover 1st edition 2016
This work is subject to copyright. All rights are reserved by the Publisher, whether the whole or part of the material is concerned, specifically the rights of translation, reprinting, reuse of illustrations, recitation, broadcasting, reproduction on microfilms or in any other physical way, and transmission or information storage and retrieval, electronic adaptation, computer software, or by similar or dissimilar methodology now known or hereafter developed.
The use of general descriptive names, registered names, trademarks, service marks, etc. in this publication does not imply, even in the absence of a specific statement, that such names are exempt from the relevant protective laws and regulations and therefore free for general use.
The publisher, the authors and the editors are safe to assume that the advice and information in this book are believed to be true and accurate at the date of publication. Neither the publisher nor the authors or the editors give a warranty, express or implied, with respect to the material contained herein or for any errors or omissions that may have been made.

Printed on acid-free paper

This Springer imprint is published by Springer Nature
The registered company is Springer International Publishing AG
The registered company address is: Gewerbestrasse 11, 6330 Cham, Switzerland

With love and appreciation to
Donna and Judy
without whose help and support,
this book would not have been possible.

Preface

Contemporary anesthesia care, like virtually all segments of medicine, requires its practitioners to adhere to evidence-based medicine in their daily practice to the maximum extent possible. This policy has the effect of both standardizing much of the care provided and presumably providing the highest quality of care. These represent distinct advantages to patients requiring anesthesia. However, neither the content nor the quality of evidence-based practice is perfect. From time to time on careful reanalysis, "best practice" is found to be flawed. Many evidence-based findings become "fact" and part of everyday practice without their ever being verified or even reanalyzed by other investigators. Understandably, scientists would rather publish "a new study with new findings" than painstakingly undertake a study to confirm what another scientific group has already reported. "Best evidence" may also be misinterpreted, applied in an inappropriate way or extended to all patient populations beyond what is justified from the data, or simply wrong. A perfect example of the latter is the fact that for years, it was believed and supported by some scientific studies that anesthesia caused long-term decline in cognitive dysfunction in the elderly. A recent study has documented the fallacy of that conclusion [1, 2]. Some have characterized strict adherence to evidence-based practice as "mindless medicine" because of bureaucratic rules that prevent deviation from a standard protocol regardless of its appropriateness for any specific patient.

As a result of the importance given to evidence-based anesthesia, practices based on experience or common sense are suspect and often denigrated. Further, some clinical practices do not lend themselves to scientific validation, as examples in this textbook will show. This is where the art of anesthesia plays an important role in maintaining the highest quality of anesthesia care.

This book is not intended to be a comprehensive textbook of anesthesiology. Rather, we have selected key topics in the specialty where we believe the art of anesthesiology has been generally overlooked, misunderstood, or forgotten. The art of anesthesia encompasses a whole host of practices that are based on long-standing, effective experiences and common sense. When combined with the science of anesthesia, the art of anesthesia gives clinicians powerful tools that will make their practices safer, more effective, and efficient and will bring greater satisfaction to their patients. The expectation is that teachers of anesthesia who use this text will find useful pearls that will enhance their teaching skills. It is expected that students of anesthesia who use this text will learn that there is an art to anesthesia and that it is reasonable or even desirable to accept and practice principles based on experiences not documented by double-blind studies and scientific validation. Just as the absence of randomized controlled trials should not preclude the use of parachutes, anesthesiologists should not limit patient care to the exclusion of common sense and clinical experience [3].

References

1. Dokkedal U, Hansen TG, Rasmussen LS, Mengel-From J, Christensen K. Cognitive functioning after surgery in middle-aged and elderly Danish twins. Anesthesiology. 2016;124:312–321.
2. Avidan MS, Evers AS. The fallacy of persistent postoperative cognitive decline. Anesthesiology. 2015;124:255–258.
3. Smith GCS, Pell JP. Parachute use to prevent death and major trauma related to gravitational challenges: systematic review of randomized controlled trials. BMJ. 2003;327:1459.

Los Angeles, CA, USA   C. Philip Larson Jr., MDCM
Stanford, CA, USA   Richard A. Jaffe, MD, PhD

Acknowledgment

Several of the chapters in this text are revisions of articles that first appeared in the publication "Current Reviews in Clinical Anesthesia." We would like to thank Dr. Frank Moya for the permission to revise and publish these articles.

Contents

Chapter 1
Preoperative Evaluation

There is both an art and a science to the preoperative evaluation of the surgical patient. The science of preoperative evaluation is well documented in all of the standard textbooks of anesthesiology. What should be included in the history and physical examination, and what laboratory studies should be performed both for routine surgical and anesthesia procedures and for special medical or surgical illnesses or special operative procedures has been described in detail. What is generally not included are suggestions or recommendations for how to make the anesthesiologist-patient encounter more effective and satisfying for both parties. This chapter is our effort to improve the preoperative evaluation experience, improve the image and confidence of patients in their anesthesia provider, lessen the chance for errors in anesthesia care because of haste or misunderstanding, and thereby lessen the chance for patient anger and a lawsuit because of a less than optimal outcome.

Telephone Consultation

One of the most effective ways for an anesthesia provider to initiate a meaningful relationship with a surgical patient is to telephone him or her the afternoon or evening before the scheduled procedure. Since today, most patients are admitted to a preoperative surgical suite on the day of scheduled surgery, there is seldom an opportunity to physically meet patients in advance of that encounter. A nurse or physician will often meet patients when they visit the preoperative anesthesia clinic, and get an initial overview of what will occur on the day of surgery. While this is helpful to patients, the specifics of the anesthesia plan cannot be discussed because these are not the personnel who will be providing the anesthetic care.

When contact is made by telephone, the anesthesiologist should identify him or herself and indicate that he/she has been requested to provide anesthesia care for the forthcoming surgery. It is always courteous to ask if this is a good time to discuss the anesthetic plan. Whenever possible, the anesthesia provider should have

© Springer International Publishing Switzerland 2017
C.P. Larson Jr., R.A. Jaffe, *Practical Anesthetic Management*,
DOI 10.1007/978-3-319-42866-6_1

reviewed all available medical records including the preoperative anesthesia clinic summary before contacting the patient. The caller may ask a few questions that amplify on material in the medical records or ask a few questions that are not included in the records, but should not discuss clearly described items. To do so makes the patient wonder if the system is incompetent when it is necessary to repeat all of the same information that was given once. In closing the encounter, the anesthesiologist should answer any questions and tell the patient when and where they will meet the next day, and that they are looking forward to taking care of him/her. Finally, the anesthesiologist should reassure the patient that he/she is in good hands, and that everything should go well tomorrow. Patients are very impressed when a physician or nurse anesthetist takes the time to telephone in advance, and when the caller is familiar with the patient's medical history. This goes a long way towards establishing rapport with the patient. Another telephone call to the patient at home a day or two after discharge from hospital to inquire about how the patient is doing postoperatively adds further to the creation of a favorable impression.

Preoperative Anesthetic Evaluation

It is absolutely essential that the anesthesia provider reviews the patient's chart in its entirety, and make note of any key issues on the preoperative anesthetic evaluation sheet or in the electronic medical record. This record is a legal document and is analyzed in microscopic detail for what it does or does not contain if an untoward event should occur as a result of anesthesia or surgery and a lawsuit is filed. Sufficient time should be taken to ensure that the record is both complete and relevant to that patient and procedure. The use of unmodified templates and preset phrases in electronic medical records may not adequately document that the anesthesiologist is aware of any patient-specific factors that will modify the anesthetic plan. Furthermore, an image of carelessness, incompetence, or indifference may be conveyed when an anesthesia provider states that he/she completed the preoperative evaluation, including filling out the evaluation form, performing a physical exam, and having the anesthesia consent signed in a time frame of 10–15 min in a complex case that goes bad. Unfortunately, this happens more often than it should.

At the outset of the meeting with a patient, the anesthesia provider must establish a working rapport with the patient. This is best done by introducing oneself and indicating what his/her role will be in the surgical or other care to be provided the patient. If family members or others are present, it is essential that the anesthesia provider ask the patient if it is all right to discuss the patient's medical history in their presence. Then the anesthesia provider should spend time learning about the patient, why they are having the operation, other operations that they have had and any adverse consequences, type of anesthesia received and outcome, any allergies, and most recent food or fluid intake. Interspersed with this fact-finding, it is appropriate to ask patients about family members, including children, where they live, type of work, special interests, etc. Getting as complete a picture of a patient as possible will allow for better planning of the operative experience as well as establishing a meaningful relationship. Most people love to talk about themselves, and doing so may put them at greater ease in this time of stress and apprehension.

In addition to the above, there are key issues that the anesthesia provider must cover in the preoperative visit. One is the anesthetic options. Options that are appropriate and available should be mentioned along with the pros and cons of each. Only then can a patient make an informed decision whether he/she should have a general or regional anesthetic, a combination of both, or monitored anesthesia care if appropriate. At some point in the preoperative evaluation, the patient should be told about the surgical team and in general what will happen from the start of anesthesia until the patient leaves the recovery room. If possible, the provider may also discuss hospital recovery and time to discharge. Finally, it is advisable to perform a brief physical examination focusing on the airway, heart, lungs and surgical site.

Anesthesia Consent

One of the shortcomings of contemporary anesthesia practice is the fact that the anesthesia consent may be incorporated in the surgical consent or presented to the patient for signature on the day of surgery. Often the consent cannot be completed in advance in the preoperative anesthesia clinic, because the staff in the clinic will not be providing the anesthetic, and cannot be specific about the anesthetic plan. To address this issue, patients are usually given an overview of anesthesia from the preoperative anesthesia clinic staff, from anesthesia brochures, and/or asked to watch a video about anesthesia. Before signing the anesthesia consent, the patient should be told that there are risks with any action taken including administering or receiving an anesthetic. The anesthesia provider should ask the patient if he/she wants to hear the risks of anesthesia. If the patient says no, or that he/she already knows them, then the response should be noted on the consent form, and proceed with having the patient sign the form and then sign as the anesthesia provider. If the patient does want to hear the risks, then they should be described briefly from the most likely (i.e.: sore throat, nausea, vomiting, etc.), which will be treated if they occur, to the rarer and highly unlikely. It would certainly be ideal if patients could have a day or two to think about the specific anesthetic plan before signing the consent, but this is rarely possible logistically. It is absolutely essential that the anesthesia provider be forthright and honest when discussing anesthesia risks with patients who are ASA III or greater because of a history of one or more conditions such as arrhythmias, myocardial infarction, congestive heart failure, type 1 diabetes, respiratory insufficiency from chronic obstructive pulmonary disease or pulmonary fibrosis, renal or hepatic insufficiency, cerebrovascular disease or morbid obesity. The risks of anesthesia in these patients are greater and must be acknowledged to the patient, while at the same time reassuring that the provider will do everything necessary to keep the patient in a stable condition during the anesthetic and surgery.

Business Card

Either at the outset or the ending of the preoperative encounter with a patient, the anesthesia provider should give the patient a business card that contains the provider's name, medical affiliation, and a contact telephone number and e-mail address. With this card the patient will know the specific name of the anesthesia provider and how to contact him/her should any questions or issues arise postoperatively. Without this, the anesthesia provider appears to some patients as a "masked bandit who comes in at the last minute, provides unknown care, and sends a large bill".

Surgeon Consultation

It is generally advisable to discuss the anesthetic and surgical plans with the surgeon in advance of going to the operating room to determine if there will be any variation from the usual routine. This is essential if this is the first or second time that the anesthesia provider has worked with the surgeon, or if the operation planned is one that the provider has not participated in with the surgeon. A mutual understanding of what is to transpire will avoid later miscommunication and errors in management.

Outside Consultations

On occasion it may be necessary for the anesthesiologist to request an outside consultation regarding, for example, pulmonary or cardiac treatment optimization before elective surgery. It is important that the consulting physician understands what exactly is being requested. Unfortunately, it is not uncommon for outside consultants to state that the patient is "ready for anesthesia" or worse, to recommend a specific type of anesthetic. The consultant should understand that their role is to comment within their area of expertise, which rarely includes the patient's suitability for anesthesia. It is often helpful to state that you are requesting the consultant's opinion regarding the pulmonary (cardiac, etc.) status of the patient, and if in their opinion as a pulmonologist (or cardiologist, etc.) further treatment could improve the patient's pulmonary (cardiac, etc.) function before surgery.

Chapter 2
Induction of General Anesthesia

General anesthesia can be induced either by intravenous injection or inhalation of anesthetic drugs. The vast majority of anesthesia providers initiate induction of anesthesia by injecting a drug, usually propofol, intravenously. The reasons that this is the preferred technique are: (a) most patients have an intravenous catheter in place prior to the start of anesthesia; and (b) the induction is rapid, effective, and allows for the prompt administration of a neuromuscular blocking drug to facilitate tracheal intubation. The downside to this method of induction is that the anesthesia provider must select a predetermined dose of propofol, and then live with the consequences. If the dose is inadequate, the provider can inject more drug. If the dose is excessive, and the patient develops hypotension from myocardial depression and vasodilation, the provider must either treat the hypotension or hope that tracheal intubation will stimulate enough catecholamine release in the patient to correct the hypotension. Unfortunately, all too often the anesthesia provider selects a "standard" dose of propofol, which, when given as a bolus may quickly decrease the blood pressure. Even if given more slowly in divided doses, patients who are hypovolemic, on antihypertensive medications or have cardiovascular disease may become hypotensive. While there are no scientific studies showing that these transient hypotensive episodes have any long-term consequences, the fact that they occur so often is of concern.

Inhalation induction of anesthesia offers several advantages over the intravenous route. First, an intravenous catheter is not necessary to initiate induction. This is an important issue because a greater number of patients who have few or no intravenous access sites are coming for surgery. Many examples can be cited including small children, patients who have had chemotherapy or multiple surgical procedures, patients with a history of substance abuse, burn patients, morbidly obese patients or those who simply do not have any discernable veins. It is disconcerting and unpleasant to watch an anesthesia provider insert a needle into a patient's skin multiple times in a futile attempt to find a vein. Not only does the patient become unhappy from the pain of the needles, but also he/she loses confidence in the skills of the provider. In addition, multiple needle sticks ruin what few veins might be available later. An inhalation induction can be done safely without the presence of

© Springer International Publishing Switzerland 2017
C.P. Larson Jr., R.A. Jaffe, *Practical Anesthetic Management*,
DOI 10.1007/978-3-319-42866-6_2

an intravenous catheter. Once the patient is surgically anesthetized via the inhalation route, what veins that do exist will stand out and make obtaining intravenous access much easier.

Second, inhalation induction is safer because the rate of induction can be tailored to the patient's responses. Induction can be accelerated by increasing the inspired anesthetic concentration and by augmenting spontaneous ventilation. If blood pressure starts to decline, the inspired concentration can be decreased. If an untoward event such as an arrhythmia or severe hypotension should occur, the inhalation drug can be turned off and hyperventilation initiated. Because the venous and tissue concentrations of the inhalation drug are minimal, the patient will emerge quickly from anesthesia. Third, the volatile drugs are complete anesthetics; they produce amnesia, analgesia, autonomic control, and some degree of muscle relaxation.

Several drugs are available for inhalation induction, but sevoflurane is by far the best drug for this purpose. It has a pleasant odor, and because of its low blood-gas solubility coefficient (0.6), the uptake will be rapid. It is not an airway irritant, so it does not promote coughing or laryngospasm during induction. Induction can be done with sevoflurane alone or in combination with nitrous oxide 50–60 %. The advantage of using nitrous oxide for a few breaths before introducing sevoflurane is that nitrous oxide is odorless and will establish a level of amnesia such that the patient will not be aware of the sevoflurane when it is introduced.

What must be done correctly to have optimum success with an inhalation induction? First, the operating room lights should be dimmed to simulate a sleeping environment, and the personnel in the room should be instructed to keep conversation and noise to a minimum until the induction is complete. Second, the mask for induction must fit reasonable snuggly to the patient's face. Substantial air entrainment under the mask will greatly delay induction. Third, the provider must use a high gas flow, approximately 10 L/min of either oxygen or a 50–50 mixture of nitrous oxide–oxygen. The reason for the high gas flow is to wash out the 7–8 L anesthetic circuit of air and replace it with anesthetic. Fourth, tell the patient to breathe as they normally do. While big deep breaths will hasten induction, it is likely that this is self-defeating unless the mask is perfectly sealed to the face. Big deep breaths generate a higher negative pressure under the mask during inhalation, and if the mask fit is not perfect, the larger transmask pressure will entrain air under the mask. Normal breathing does not generate more than 1–2 cmH$_2$O transmask pressure difference, so air entrainment will be minimal. In daily clinical practice the mask-face seal is seldom perfect.

Within 2–3 min of the start of the inhalation induction it is possible to initiate assisted ventilation to augment tidal volume and accelerate the induction. Very soon thereafter the anesthesia provider can transition to controlled ventilation. Thus by regulating the inspired gas mixture and ventilation the anesthesia provider can regulate the rate of induction of anesthesia. Even in patients with venous access there may be no safer way to induce anesthesia in the presence of co-morbidities of concern, unstable vital signs, or hypovolemic from blood loss or dehydration. The induction progresses much more smoothly if the anesthesia provider talks to the patient continuously during the induction. The provider should give the patient specific instructions to breathe in and out and not to move his/her arms or legs. If these instructions are repeated over and over, the patient will transition through the excitement stage of induction uneventfully. Once the patient is anesthetized, the provider can either intubate the trachea quickly or insert an LMA and allow the patient to breathe spontaneously or place the patient on controlled ventilation. At that juncture, the provider can step aside and establish intravenous access or ask a colleague to do so.

There have been a number of studies comparing intravenous inductions with propofol with inhalation inductions with sevoflurane. The inhalation inductions varied, some using 8% sevoflurane with [1–3] or without [4, 5] nitrous oxide, some using a vital capacity induction [1, 3], and others studying the comparison in elderly [3] or hypertensive patients [6]. Patient acceptance of inhalation induction depended on several factors including the technique used, fear of needle sticks, etc. In general, when performed smoothly and efficiently, most patients found inhalation induction anesthesia acceptable and in some cases preferable.

Summary

Every anesthesia provider needs to know how to perform an inhalation induction of anesthesia in adults as well children in an efficient, effective, safe manner. It is a technique that is not rigorously taught in training programs, and consequently not widely used in community or university practices. Many question whether adult patients will willingly accept an inhalation induction. Those patients who have endured multiple, painful needle sticks in an attempt to find a vein readily embrace the technique and frequently ask why other anesthesia providers have not offered it to them. Both the scientific and anecdotal evidence indicates that inhalation inductions are more widely accepted by patients than most anesthesia providers realize.

References

1. Philip BK, Lombard L, Roaf ER, Drager LR, Calalang I, Philip JH. Comparison of vital capacity induction with sevoflurane to intravenous induction with propofol for adult ambulatory patients. Anesth Analg. 1999;89:623.
2. Jellish WS, Lien CA, Fontenot H, Jerrel H, Hall R. The comparison effects of sevoflurane versus propofol in the induction and maintenance of anesthesia in adult patients. Anesth Analg. 1996;82:479–85.
3. van den Berg AA, Chitty DA, Jones RD, Sohel MS, Shahen A. Intravenous or inhaled induction of anesthesia in adults? An audit of preoperative patient preferences. Anesth Analg. 2005;100:1422–4.
4. Walpole R, Logan M. Effect of sevoflurane concentration on inhalation induction of anesthesia in the elderly. Br J Anaesth. 1999;82:20–4.
5. Thwaites A, Edmends S, Smith I. Inhalation induction with sevoflurane: a double-blind comparison with propofol. Br J Anaesth. 1997;78:356–61.
6. Nathan N, Vial G, Benrhaiem M, Peyclit A, Feiss P. Induction with propofol target-concentration infusion vs. 8% sevoflurane inhalation and alfentanil in hypertensive patients. Anaesthesia. 2001;56:251–7.

Chapter 3
Role of the Laryngeal Mask Airway in Airway Management

There are multiple ways that a laryngeal mask airway (LMA) can be used to facilitate airway management, and in some circumstances will be a lifesaving instrument.

Uses of an LMA in Airway Management
- Substitute for bag-mask ventilation
- Alternative to endotracheal tube
- Aid in nasal intubation
- Conduit for fiberoptic intubation
- Conduit for "blind" oral intubation
- Establishing emergency airway

Since development of the "classic" LMA by Brain, there have been a number of modifications in design, but for the most part their function is similar to the original. The "classic" LMA has an inflatable mask design that fits over the glottic opening to lessen the risk of gastric distension with positive pressure ventilation. An alternative design utilizes a supraglottic balloon to prevent gastric distension with positive pressure ventilation. The KingLT(S) LMA has two conduit tubes, one for ventilation and the other through which an orogastric tube can be inserted for suction and decompression of the stomach (Fig. 3.1).

In any consideration of the use of a LMA, the issue of its application in a patient with a potential full stomach always arises. To dispense with this issue at the outset, it would almost always be better to go directly to placement of an endotracheal tube in patients with a potential full stomach who require general anesthesia. In the relatively rare circumstances where an LMA is needed in the presence of a potential full stomach, for example as a conduit for a difficult tracheal intubation, other precautions can be taken. The options would include decompressing the stomach with an

© Springer International Publishing Switzerland 2017
C.P. Larson Jr., R.A. Jaffe, *Practical Anesthetic Management*,
DOI 10.1007/978-3-319-42866-6_3

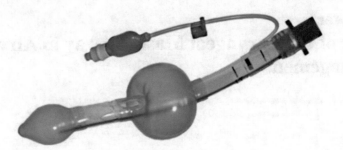

Fig. 3.1 Multiple use, sterilizable KingLT(S) with ventilation and gastric access channels. Two balloons, one positioned in the esophagus and the other in the oropharynx isolate the airway. Both balloons are inflated from a single injection port. It also comes as a single use, disposable device [KingLT(S)-D]. Picture courtesy of Ambu, Inc.

Fig. 3.2 I-gel. Courtesy of
Intersurgical Complete
Respiratory Systems

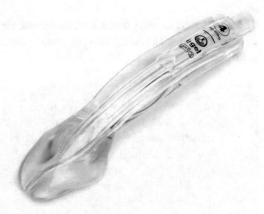

oro- or nasogastric tube with the patient awake and then maintaining firm cricoid pressure from the induction of anesthesia and insertion of the LMA until the endotracheal tube is in place and the tube cuff inflated. Another option would be to topicalize the oropharynx, but not the trachea, with local anesthetic, and then under light sedation insert a KingLT(S) or similar supraglottic airway that incorporates a conduit for inserting a gastric tube, which can be used to decompress the stomach before instituting cricoid pressure and inducing general anesthesia.

The recently developed I-gel has become increasingly popular in clinical practice because of its simplicity in design, ease of insertion, and effectiveness as a supraglottic airway (Fig. 3.2) [1, 2]. Unlike other supraglottic airways, the I-gel does not have an inflatable cuff. Rather, it has a gel-like frame composed of a thermoplastic elastomer, which when warmed in the oropharynx molds to fit the laryngeal structures. As it warms, it provides a progressively firmer seal with the laryngeal opening so manual or mechanical ventilation is safe and effective. Prewarming the I-gel to 42° before insertion facilitates both ease of insertion and time to laryngeal seal [3].

Uses of an LMA in Airway Management

As a Substitute for Bag-Mask Ventilation

This is one of the most useful and frequent uses of an LMA in airway management. Many short surgical cases, which in the past would have been managed by bag-mask ventilation, can more easily be managed with an LMA, thereby freeing the hands of the anesthesia provider to do other things such as charting, drawing up drugs, etc. This has, in turn, increased both the efficiency and effectiveness of the anesthesia provider (Fig. 3.3).

As a Substitute for an Endotracheal Tube

This use has truly revolutionized the practice of general anesthesia. In the past, operations lasting more than an hour, or operations about the head, neck, upper thorax or arms would generally require insertion of an endotracheal tube to ensure an adequate airway during the operative procedure. Now, many of these operations can be performed safely utilizing an LMA for airway management. Is there any operative duration beyond which it is inappropriate to use an LMA? Some practitioners are reluctant to use an LMA for operations expected to last for more than 2–3 h,

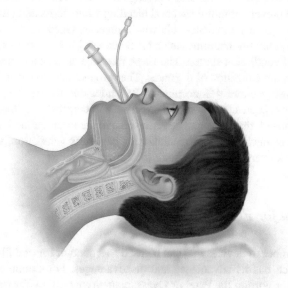

Fig. 3.3 Proper positioning of a laryngeal mask airway (LMA)

primarily because of the concern for the development of progressive pulmonary atelectasis. However, there are no scientific studies that clearly document that three or more hours of spontaneous breathing via an LMA result in greater atelectasis than would occur under the same circumstances with an endotracheal tube in place. Other practitioners are reluctant to use an LMA if the operative procedure requires the use of a neuromuscular blocking drug. The concern here is that prolonged manual or mechanical ventilation may result in gastric distension resulting in such complications as regurgitation of gastric fluid, elevation of the diaphragm and resultant loss of lung volume, or gastric rupture. However, again there is no scientific evidence that gastric distension of any consequence will occur if the airway pressure does not exceed 20–25 cmH$_2$O, regardless of how long mechanical ventilation is utilized.

For Airway Management During Nasal Fiberoptic Intubation

A wide variety of operations about the face, jaw or upper airway require the use of a nasotracheal tube for airway management. Generally, this intubation is performed with the patient surgically anesthetized, both for patient comfort and for ease of insertion. The intubation can be completed using a nasal fiberoptic scope, or under direct laryngoscopy using a Magill forceps. Regardless of which technique is used, it is imperative to topicalize the nasal passage before insertion of the scope or the tracheal tube to prevent or minimize nasal bleeding while performing the intubation. Use of an LMA greatly facilitates this whole process. Once general anesthesia is instituted and preferably neuromuscular blockade established, an LMA is inserted and mechanical ventilation started. The LMA frees the anesthesia provider's hands to proceed with topicalization of the nares. The provider can do a careful, thorough topicalization using either 4 % cocaine or 2 % lidocaine to which epinephrine or phenylephrine has been added to obtain effective vasoconstriction. Once the topicalization is completed, the LMA can be removed and the nasal intubation performed. This technique is much superior to maintaining bag-mask ventilation, and having to remove the mask every time the operator topicalizes the nares.

As a Conduit for Fiberoptic Intubation

There are a number of devices that can be used as a conduit for oral fiberoptic intubation, and each has its advantages and disadvantages. For example, because of their open center portion the Patel or Ovassapian airways allow for removal of the airway after insertion of the endotracheal tube (Fig. 3.4). However, these airways have two drawbacks. One, they are often too short so that the distal end of the airway generally does not place the scope at the glottic opening; and two, they are

Fig. 3.4 Ovassapian
airway. Image courtesy of
the Wood Library-Museum
of Anesthesiology,
Schaumburg, Illinois

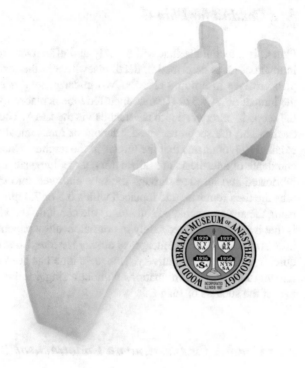

white in color which makes distinguishing the airway from the tongue and surrounding soft tissue difficult for those inexperienced in fiberoptics. The Tudor-
Williams (pink) airway overcomes both of those disadvantages, but the 15 mm
connector on the tube must be removed before the airway can be removed from the
mouth after insertion of the tube.

The classic LMA is an excellent conduit for oral fiberoptic intubation. When
properly placed, the tip of the LMA is directly in front of the glottic opening, and
the characteristic color makes it easy to distinguish when the scope leaves the LMA
channel. The number 4 LMA is the ideal size for most adults, although a number 3
functions well in smaller adults or those with deformed upper airways due to disease, prior surgery in the mouth or neck, or a short thyromental distance. The number 5 LMA should rarely be used as a conduit regardless of patient size because
when properly placed it frequently invaginates the epiglottis making it impossible
to see the glottic opening. The disposable LMA's are also not recommended because
of their translucent color, which makes it hard to distinguish LMA tube from patient
tissue. The disposable LMA's may also have a flange at the distal end of the conduit,
which serves as an obstruction when advancing a tracheal tube after proper placement of the scope. If necessary, this flange can be cut out with a pair of scissors
before inserting the LMA in the mouth.

As a Conduit for Plan C

Plan C is a technique that will quickly and effectively resolve almost all difficult intubations. It is described in detail elsewhere in the text (Chap. 4). Basically, the plan involves inserting a classic LMA under general anesthesia as the conduit for the intubation. A 5.5 or 6.0 mm uncuffed tube is placed over a fiberoptic scope, and the scope is introduced into the trachea via the LMA. The tube is advanced into the trachea and the scope removed. Manual or mechanical ventilation with return of exhaled CO_2 confirms that the tube is in the trachea. Once ventilation, oxygenation and depth of anesthesia are satisfactory, a medium size airway exchange catheter is lubricated and inserted through the tube and well into the trachea. The LMA and tube are then removed and replaced with a 6.5 or 7.0 mm cuffed endotracheal tube, using the airway exchange catheter as the conduit. The advantage of this technique is that it can be practiced safely in normal, healthy patients, so that when a difficult intubation occurs, or an emergency airway is needed, one can perform the technique quickly, safely, and effectively. This technique has been used in hundreds of cases known to be difficult intubations without a single failure. The LMA is an integral part of the success of Plan C.

As a Conduit for Inserting an Endotracheal Tube

Several LMA's have been designed to allow for direct insertion of an endotracheal tube as a "blind" procedure. The most widely used ones are the LMA Fastrach™ or Fastrach™ single use (Fig. 3.5). These devices have a unique curvature with a handle for lifting it while inserting the endotracheal tube. Generally, intubation is more successful if one uses the largest LMA Fastrach that can be inserted into the mouth. The number 5 is preferred in most adults, with the number 4 being used in smaller adults. With the patient anesthetized and preferably paralyzed, the LMA is inserted and manual or mechanical ventilation started. While lifting gently on the handle, a special, silicone rubber endotracheal tube is inserted through the LMA into the trachea. Attaching the 15 mm connector on the tube to the anesthesia circuit and visualizing exhaled CO_2 confirms proper placement. The 15 mm connector is removed and a specialized pusher is inserted inside the tube. The LMA is then removed while holding to the tube in place with the pusher. The 15 mm connector is then reinserted on the tube and attached to the anesthesia circuit. While a useful device, the intubating LMA is not ideal in emergency situation for several reasons. First, the technique is not uniformly successful in difficult or even normal airways. Second, multiple attempts may be necessary, each of which may consume valuable time. One cause for failure is that the tip of the LMA may be invaginating the epiglottis over the glottic opening thereby preventing the tube from going into the trachea. Lateral rotation of the LMA may resolve this problem.

Third, since the tracheal tube is reusable, the cuff on the tube must be tested for leaks prior to insertion. And fourth, one must ensure that the reusable tube has been

Fig. 3.5 Disposable
Fastrach LMA. Picture
courtesy of Ambu, Inc.

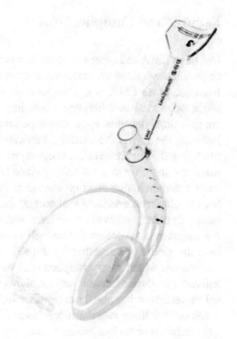

properly cleaned and sterilized prior to use. If two or three attempts at tracheal intubation with the LMA Fastrach are unsuccessful, it is advisable to remove the Fastrach and insert a classic LMA for performing fiberoptic intubation instead of attempting it through the Fastrach. The extreme curvature of the Fastrach makes fiberoptic intubation needlessly difficult. Other LMA's designed as a conduit for insertion of an endotracheal tube are less curved in structure than the LMA Fastrach, but work in a similar manner. A standard endotracheal tube can be used with these. The LMA CTrach™ is similar to the LMA Fastrach except that it has a fiberoptic channel and light source at the distal end that are attached to a small external video screen. This system allows for direct visualization of the glottic opening as the tube is inserted. However, the picture is small and identification of the glottis can be difficult. Use of this device requires some training and experience.

As an Emergency Airway in the Field

Because of its ease of insertion and minimal risk of injury, the LMA is an ideal device for use by emergency medical personnel when an airway needs to be established in the field or even in a medical clinic or hospital setting. If the insertion is difficult, trauma to the hard palate may occur, but the attendant bleeding is usually minimal and the injury of no lasting importance. Insertion may also precipitate laryngospasm, but this is easily resolved with the laryngospasm maneuver (see Chap. 5).

Failures and Complications

Use of an LMA and other supraglottic airways is not without failures and complications, although these are uncommon or even rare. The most common complication from use of an LMA is a postoperative sore throat. Usually it is associated with slight or modest oropharyngeal bleeding during insertion. The incidence of this complication depends upon the experience and skill of the anesthesia provider inserting the LMA. Presumably, lubrication of the LMA cuff and gentle insertion following the curvature of the oropharynx will minimize this problem. Another failure is the inability to position any sized LMA in the center of the oropharynx and have it remain in that position instead of falling off to one side. In this position it is hard to obtain an adequate seal around the glottic opening. This occurs most commonly in elderly edentulous patients with a slack jaw and redundant soft tissue in the oropharynx. Another failure will occur if the LMA invaginates the epiglottis over the glottic opening thereby impairing both spontaneous and positive pressure ventilation. Much rarer complications include sialadenopathy or swelling of the salivary glands and nerve injury involving the lingual, glossopharyngeal, hypoglossal or recurrent laryngeal nerves. For lack of any other explanation, it has been assumed that these rare neuropraxias are due to pressure from the LMA cuff from over inflation or malpositioning. Once the LMA is in place and functioning well, it is advisable to deflate the LMA cuff just to the point a slight leak is prevented, although there is no evidence that doing so would prevent the rare injuries.

Video Laryngoscopy

Recently it has been proposed that video laryngoscopy should be the new standard of care for tracheal intubation [4]. It also has been suggested that video laryngoscopy has all but eliminated the need for direct laryngoscopy. In a 2009 study of experienced anesthesiologists comparing the Glidescope, the Pentax AWS and a Macintosh laryngoscope on simulated difficult airways, the Pentax scope was judged easiest to use, providing the best view of the glottis and the shortest time to successful intubation (Fig. 3.6) [5]. The findings in this study need to be confirmed by a similar study in patients known to be difficult intubations. A systematic review and meta-analysis comparing video and direct laryngoscopic techniques concluded that direct laryngoscopy provided an inferior view of the glottis without affecting successful first attempt intubation [6]. Indeed, most studies suggest that in experienced hands there is no significance difference in intubation success rates between direct and video laryngoscopy. We would argue that the skills necessary to become adept at the use of a Glidescope or similar device do not translate into the skills necessary to manage the truly difficult airway. When video laryngoscopic techniques fail the patient will be best served by an anesthesiologist well practiced in alternative airway management techniques.

Fig. 3.6 Pentax
laryngoscope courtesy of
Richards Medical
Equipment Inc.

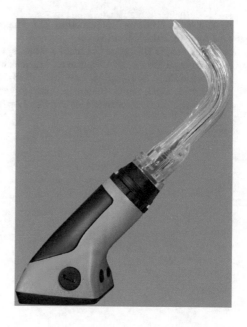

Summary

The LMA and other supraglottic airways have proven to be invaluable tools for accomplishing safe, effective airway management. The classic or disposable LMA, or the I-gel in multiple sizes should be immediately available in the workstation of every anesthesia provider who is responsible for providing general or regional anesthesia to patients. It is an excellent device for instituting an effective airway in emergencies. It is also a perfect conduit for performing fiberoptic intubation. The LMA is integral to the management of patients who are known or suspected to have a difficult airway due to either difficult bag-mask ventilation or difficult intubation. Proper use of an LMA should eliminate the need for multiple attempts at direct laryngoscopy, a course of management that is fraught with life-threatening risks.

References

1. Levitan RM, Kinkle WC. Initial anatomic investigations of the I-gel airway: a novel supraglottic airway without inflatable cuff. Anaesthesia. 2005;60:1022–6.
2. Leventis C, Chalkias A, Sampanis M, Foulidou X, Xanthos T. Emergency airway management by paramedics: comparison between standard endotracheal intubation, laryngeal mask airway, and I-gel. Eur J Emerg Med. 2014;21:371–3.
3. Komasawa N, Nishihara I, Tatsumi S, Minami T. Prewarming of the I-gel facilitates successful insertion and ventilation efficacy with muscle relaxation: a randomized study. J Clin Anesth. 2014;26:663–7.

4. Zaouter C, Calderon J, Hemmerling TM. Videolaryngoscopy as a new standard of care. Br J Anaesth. 2015;114(2):181–3.
5. Malik MA, O'Donoghue C, Carney J, Maharaj CH, Harte BH, Laffey JG. Comparison of the Glidescope, the Pentax AWS, and the Macintosh laryngoscope in experienced anaesthetists: a manikin study. Br J Anaesth. 2009;102(1):128–34.
6. Griesdale DEG, Liu D. Glidescope video-laryngoscopy vs. direct laryngoscopy for endotracheal intubation: a systematic review. Can J Anesth. 2012;59:41–52.

Chapter 4
Essentials of Airway Management

Management of the airway is **the most important technical skill** expected of an anesthesiologist. No one in medicine has the responsibility for managing the panoply of airway problems that the anesthesiologist encounters in the course of providing surgical anesthesia or critical care medicine. ENT surgeons may be effective in managing certain airway problems, but they do not have the training or breadth of experience to deal with the full spectrum of airway abnormalities that anesthesiologists need to address. When one of us first started in anesthesia 53 years ago there were only three ways the airway was managed during surgery or during a cardiac arrest: bag-mask ventilation; standard endotracheal intubation; or blind nasotracheal intubation. Now we have an abundance of tools with which to tackle the normal or difficult airway. Many in our specialty believe that the anesthesiologist should be reasonably skilled with most of the techniques available, stating that "the more arrows that you have in your quiver, the more effective you will be". While an interesting idea, that concept is flawed. The reason is simple. To maintain an effective level of skill with any airway technique, it must be practiced on a regular basis. Studies indicate that the incidence of encountering a difficult airway ranges between 5 and 10 % of all surgical patients depending upon the type of surgical practice. If the average anesthesiologist does 600 cases a year, he/she would encounter 30–60 difficult airway patients in a year or about one patient every 1 or 2 weeks. That is too small a patient population to consider trying to become expert in all of the available airway techniques. Instead, we recommend that the anesthesiologist become skilled with a select number of techniques that are reliable, effective, safe, and can be practiced in normal patients, so that when the difficult airway suddenly arises, the provider can be confident that one of the practiced techniques will be successful in establishing an airway. This chapter will highlight those airway techniques that we believe will successfully overcome almost any airway difficulty.

Electronic supplementary material: The online version of this chapter (doi:10.1007/978-3-319-42866-6_4) contains supplementary material, which is available to authorized users. Videos can also be accessed at http://link.springer.com/chapter/10.1007/978-3-319-42866-6_4.

© Springer International Publishing Switzerland 2017
C.P. Larson Jr., R.A. Jaffe, *Practical Anesthetic Management*,
DOI 10.1007/978-3-319-42866-6_4

Evaluation of the Airway (Video 4.1.)

The first and most important step in airway management is to assess the airway in terms of difficulty for either bag-mask ventilation or endotracheal intubation. Conditions that make for difficult bag-mask ventilation are uncommon and generally obvious from the history and physical examination. The only exception would be lingual tonsillar hyperplasia, which may not be easily detected during routine oral examination. However, this condition is not of great concern since the evidence indicates that the lungs of patients with this condition can be readily ventilated with an LMA. In contrast, difficulty with tracheal intubation using standard laryngoscopy is not as predictable despite many proposed methods for evaluating the airway. Because ability to intubate the trachea using standard laryngoscopy is not highly predictable, it is important that the laryngoscopist have **alternative means at hand**, particularly if there is any suspicion that the intubation may be difficult.

Conditions Making Bag-Mask Ventilation Difficult
1. Poor mask fit due to facial distortion, facial trauma, heavy, thick beard
2. Mass (tumor, infection) in oropharynx, larynx
3. Edentulous mouth, large tongue
4. Obese neck, redundant jowls
5. Mediastinal mass compressing the trachea
6. Radiation therapy to face, neck, or mediastinum
7. Fractured larynx
8. Compromised lung volume from abdominal mass, thoracic trauma, pneumothorax
9. Lingual tonsillar hyperplasia (easily resolved with an LMA)

Preoperative Assessment for Difficult Intubation
1. History from patient or records of a difficult intubation
2. Ability to open mouth
3. Size of tongue and central incisors
4. Mallampati score
5. Thyromental distance <5 cm
6. Length and thickness of neck
7. Range of motion of head and neck
8. Upper lip bite test

Preoxygenation

Preoxygenation of the patient's lungs is an important first step in managing the airway. To do it quickly and effectively the provider must establish a tight mask fit, utilize a gas flow of oxygen of about 10 L/min to wash out air from the anesthesia circuit (up to 8 L volume) and the patient's FRC (adult about 2 L). If the mask fit is tight, deep breathing by the patient will hasten the elimination of nitrogen from the patient's lungs, but if it is not tight, normal breathing by the patient is preferred because it generates a lower transmask pressure gradient and is thus less likely to entrain air. The goal is not only to replace the nitrogen in the lungs with oxygen, but also to increase the quantity of dissolved oxygen in the plasma. At a PaO_2 of 100 mmHg, the blood carries about 0.3 mL oxygen/100 mL plasma, while at a PaO_2 of 500 mmHg the blood carries about 1.5 mL oxygen/100 mL plasma. Estimating that the average adult has about 3500 mL plasma, the quantity of oxygen in the blood increases from about 10 mL to more than 50 mL, which provides additional oxygen at the tissue level. For practical purposes, when the expired oxygen concentration in the exhaled gas mixture reaches 80–85 %, preoxygenation is complete. How much "safe time" preoxygenation provides depends upon multiple factors but most importantly the cardiac output and the patient's body habitus as it affects FRC. The greater the cardiac output or the larger the abdominal volume (smaller FRC), the shorter the safe time before the oxygen saturation begins to decrease. A recent study found that using high oxygen concentrations (>80 %) during preoxygenation resulted in a greater degree of basal atelectasis than when lower (<40 %) oxygen concentrations were used [1]. However, there was no documented risk associated with the greater atelectasis, and the authors concluded that the traditional practice of using high oxygen concentration during preoxygenation should be continued because of the longer time to desaturation that it affords. They also recommended the use of end expiratory positive pressure during induction to minimize the development of atelectasis.

Bag-Mask Ventilation

Confirming that bag-mask ventilation is possible is an important step in the airway management of any patient undergoing general anesthesia. Conditions predisposing to difficult or impossible bag-mask ventilation are few in number, and generally highly predictable from the preoperative assessment (above). If there is any question in the anesthesiologist's mind about the ability to perform bag-mask ventilation in a patient, then inducing general anesthesia with intravenous agents (i.e.: propofol) should be done very cautiously or not at all. The safest, most conservative approach is to establish the airway with the patient awake using fiberoptic laryngoscopy. This technique will be described later in the text. The other option is to perform an inhalation induction with sevoflurane-oxygen. Whenever possible we prefer this latter technique because of its applicability, simplicity and safety. It can be extremely difficult and even impossible in some patients, especially smokers, to diminish the gag or cough reflexes to the point that one is able to accomplish an awake fiberoptic intubation. Hence an asleep fiberoptic intubation is the only alternative. If as the inspired concentration of sevoflurane is increased the patient develops difficulty with ventilation or airway obstruction that cannot be readily resolved with a jaw thrust, oral or nasal airway or LMA insertion, then turning off the sevoflurane with its low blood:gas partition coefficient will allow the patient to wake up very quickly because of the minimal tissue level of sevoflurane. One can then resort to awake fiberoptic intubation. If airway patency remains intact during inhalation induction, instituting manual ventilation as soon as possible will greatly speed up the induction process. Once the patient is in a surgical plane of anesthesia, fiberoptic intubation can be accomplished with or without muscle relaxant using an LMA or oral airway (Patel, Ovassapian, or Tudor-Williams) as a conduit.

Standard Endotracheal Intubation (Plan A) (Video 4.2)

Most anesthesiologists learn endotracheal intubation primarily by trial and error, and as a result develop habits that make successful intubation less likely when encountering a difficult airway. Whenever possible it is important to optimize patient positioning before beginning tracheal intubation. Unfortunately, these simple conditions are often forgotten, and consequently intubation is made more difficult than it need be. The patient's head should always be at the very top of the operating table or bed so the operator does not have to reach forward to get to the mouth. If the surgeon needs the patient in another position on the bed, the patient can always be moved after the tracheal intubation is completed. The table or bed height should be at the operator's umbilical level so that the operator does not have to bend over during the intubation. The operator should stand at a 45° angle to the patient's right, i.e. facing the right wall (Fig. 4.1), which allows the operator to rest his/her elbow against the left hip or thorax. With the left arm acting only as a fulcrum (no lifting or pushing), the operator shifts weight from the back foot to the front foot and the direction of movement of the laryngoscope is along the plane of the handle. This maneuver lifts the patient's head into the sniff position for optimum visualization.

Since all of the lifting of the head is done with the flat surface of the McIntosh or straight blade, there is no injury to the soft tissues of the oropharynx. Most importantly, this technique converts endotracheal intubation from a left arm activity, which is now entirely passive, to a leg activity, where most laryngoscopists' strength lies. Before starting intubation, the endotracheal tube should be lubricated and placed high in the laryngoscopist's left axilla. Once the laryngeal opening is visualized, the laryngoscopist can reach up and remove the tube from its package without ever looking away from the larynx. This is the only tube location that we have found where the average laryngoscopist does not have to look away to find the tube. Since the first endoscopic look, once established, is always the best, the operator does not want to look away to find the endotracheal tube and then look back at the larynx to discover that his/her original view is lost. The laryngoscopist should always use the smallest appropriate tube (7.0 men, 6.5–7.0 women) since smaller tubes are always easier to insert than larger tubes. If a larger tube is needed for surgical purposes, the tube can always be changed using an airway exchange catheter. This standard laryngoscopic approach is called **Plan A**.

The gold standard for determining that the tube is in the trachea and not the esophagus is by visualizing sustained end-tidal carbon dioxide on capnography.

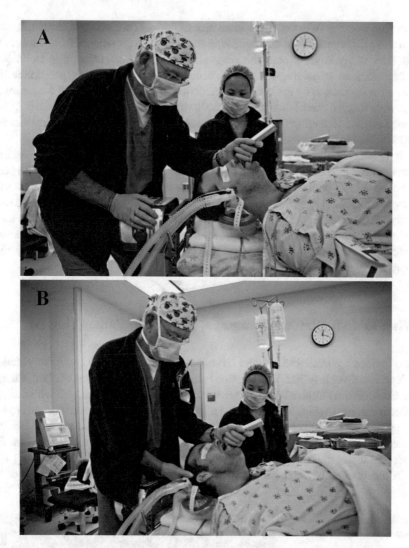

Fig. 4.1 (**a**) Incorrect posture during standard tracheal intubation. (**b**) Proper posture for standard tracheal intubation, with tracheal tube positioned in the left axilla

However, a quicker and very reliable technique is to attach the endotracheal tube to the circle system and give the patient a large breath from the reservoir bag with the tube cuff still deflated. If the tube is in the trachea, a characteristic sound emanates from the mouth, which is best described as the soft sound of wind blowing through the trees, while if the tube is in the esophagus, the sound is distinctly gurgley. Once one learns to use this test, it becomes quick and easy to discern whether the tube is in the trachea or esophagus. In the absence of capnography, one can also look for vapor or mist inside the tube with exhalation, and of course one can auscultate the chest and stomach. We don't put a great deal of faith or confidence in chest ausculta-tion as a primary means of distinguishing tracheal from esophageal intubation, hav-ing seen many cases where the diagnosis was incorrect using this technique. Experienced anesthesiologists can also usually distinguish the tube position in the trachea or esophagus by the very characteristic difference in the feel of the reservoir bag with manual ventilation. Finally, balloting the endotracheal tube cuff in the sternal notch and feeling the pilot balloon for volume changes will confirm that the endotracheal tube is in the trachea and not endobronchial or esophageal.

It is very important to limit the number of attempts at direct laryngoscopy because each attempt increases the likelihood of converting the situation from "can ventilate—can't intubate" to "can't ventilate—can't intubate". With each attempt there are increased secretions and possibly blood in the oropharynx, increased oro-pharyngeal edema, and deterioration of the anesthetic state, all of which make intu-bation and ventilation more difficult. An experienced laryngoscopist should know within one or two attempts at direct laryngoscopy whether intubation by that approach is possible.

What to do if Direct Laryngoscopy (Plan A) Fails; (Plan B)

Two options are available if direct laryngoscopy fails, and they can be used either independently or together. These options are known as **Plan B**. One method is using the Cook (Frova) Intubating catheter which is a solid, firm 70 cm tube with a slight inflection at its tip (Fig. 4.2) (Video 4.3). To use this catheter one must be able to see the epiglottis or even better the posterior portion of the arytenoid cartilages. Placing the catheter in the center of the epiglottis and dropping the hand down toward the floor will direct the catheter upward into the trachea. One can tell immediately if it is in the trachea by advancing it. If it is in the trachea, the catheter cannot be

Fig. 4.2 Straight and manually curved Cook (Frova) catheters. If catheter is to be used with the GlideScope, catheter must be curved to same shape as GlideScope blade and shape maintained during insertion into glottic opening. Courtesy of Verathon Medical

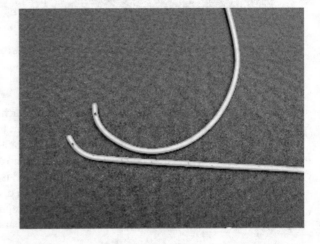

advanced easily beyond the carina, which is usually 30–40 cm in adults because of the distal inflection, while if it is in the esophagus, it can be advanced until the distal tip is at the lips. Some say that they can feel the tracheal rings as the catheter is inserted, but we find that of limited value. Once the Cook catheter is in position, an endotracheal tube can be inserted over the catheter using gentle pressure while turning the tube counterclockwise to direct its tip toward the midline. The operator will feel a slight bump as the tube passes the vocal cords. A 6.0 OD or larger tube can be inserted over the Cook catheter, but it is advisable to use as small a tracheal tube as is feasible. For most adult patients, a 7.0 OD tube is large enough to provide effective ventilation. Inserting the Cook catheter relatively blindly is safe because the catheter tip is small (5 mm OD), round and flexible. It would be difficult to perforate soft tissue during its insertion.

The other alternative in **Plan B** is to use a video laryngoscope, for example, the GlideScope®, with its high-resolution color camera in the laryngoscope blade, which transmits a video output to a detached screen (Video 4.4). Disposable blades are available in several sizes. Brightness, color and contrast are adjustable so the picture is very clear and detailed. The GlideScope® comes with a rigid stylet that is curved to match the curve of the laryngoscope blade. Unfortunately, the stylet will not fit tubes smaller than a 6.5. One can use other stylets, but they must be bent to the same shape as the blade, and they must be rigid enough to maintain their shape during insertion of the styletted tube into the trachea. As the styletted tube is inserted in the mouth and advanced into the oropharynx, the operator should initially **watch the tube, not the screen**. Failure to do this may result in inadvertent perforation of soft tissue in the oropharynx as the tube is advanced into the oral cavity. There are several case reports documenting this complication. Once the styletted tube reaches the glottic opening, it is usually necessary to withdraw the stylet 4–5 cm to allow the tube to advance further into the glottis. The Cook catheter can be used in combination with the GlideScope® provided the Cook catheter is flexed so that it has a curve that mirrors the curve of the GlideScope® blade (Video 4.5). While inserting the Cook catheter into the oropharynx, it is vital not to let it hit any structures such that it loses its shape. Using the GlideScope®, Cook catheter, or a combination of the two, tracheal intubation will be accomplished quickly and effectively in most patients who present as a difficult intubation. However, if both techniques fail for whatever reason, then the anesthesiologist should move on to Plan C.

What to do if Both Plan A and Plan B Fail (Plan C) (Video 4.6)

Plan C is the technique of choice if Plans A and B have failed, or as the primary choice in selected circumstances such as a patient with a cervical spine injury or with a known mass in the neck or throat that impairs normal ventilation. While many anesthesiologists would opt for an awake fiberoptic intubation in such patients, Plan C will accomplish the intubation safely, and in the process is quicker and easier on both patient and anesthesiologist than awake intubation. The technique of inhalation induction is described above under bag-mask ventilation.

Once the patient is anesthetized either by intravenous or preferably inhalation induction, and muscle relaxation is obtained by use of a non-depolarizing agent such as rocuronium, an LMA (#3 or 4 for women; #4 for men) is inserted. We would not recommend using the #5 LMA, even in the largest men, because it tends to invaginate the epiglottis over the laryngeal opening, making it virtually impossible to identify the laryngeal opening and insert the scope through it. The classic LMA is preferred over a disposable LMA because of its distinctive color when introducing the fiberoptic laryngoscope. If an LMA is not available or cannot be seated properly, a Tudor-Williams (#9 or 10) or other airway can be substituted and used as a conduit (Video 4.7). Mechanical ventilation is then instituted which optimizes oxygenation, ventilation and anesthetic depth with a volatile agent, and frees up the anesthesiologist's hands to proceed with the next step. Five items are needed for Plan C: an oral conduit (LMA, oral airway); a fiberoptic bronchoscope; an uncuffed tube 6.0; a medium sized airway exchange catheter (AEC 5.0 mm OD); and the final endotracheal tube (either 6.5 or 7.0 OD). The closer the final tube approximates the diameter of the AEC, the easier its insertion will be. The 6.0 uncuffed tube, with its connector **firmly attached**, is placed over the fiberoptic scope making certain that the scope does not go through the Murphy eye, and lightly taped in place at the proximal end of the scope (Video 4.8). The scope is then introduced into the conduit and advanced into the glottis opening. The distal end of the 6.0 tube is lubricated with lidocaine jelly and guided into the glottis via the scope. The scope is then removed while holding the 6.0 tube firmly in place. The 6.0 tube is then attached to the anesthetic circuit, and ventilation and oxygenation established for a second time. A high gas flow is needed to maintain ventilation because of the large gas leak between the tube and the conduit (LMA). Once ventilation, oxygenation and anesthetic depth are satisfactory, the AEC tip is lubricated and inserted through the uncuffed tube. Some resistance is met when the AEC reaches the distal end of the tube (usually about 30 cm), and may require firm insertion beyond that point while rotating the 6.0 tube without removing it. With a little practice, inserting the AEC beyond the tip of the tube becomes easy. The AEC is then advanced about 2–2.5 in. (4–6 cm) to prevent its removal from the airway with removal of the conduit and the 6.0 tube. The final tube is inserted over the AEC, again making certain that it does not go through the Murphy eye. With the AEC in the right corner of the mouth the final tube is inserted into the mouth via the AEC and rotating it counterclockwise toward the midline gently advanced into the trachea while holding the AEC still. If the tube does not advance easily, it may be either that the patient's vocal cords are not paralyzed and consequently are opening and closing, or too much of the AEC was inserted and a portion of it is curled up in the oropharynx. Pulling back slightly on the AEC will correct the latter problem. Once the final tube is in place, the AEC is removed and ventilation established.

Plan C has several major advantages. As with Plan A and B, Plan C can be practiced as often as desired on healthy, normal patients without concern for injury, so that when it is needed in a difficult intubation, the anesthesiologist has confidence that he/she can perform the task without fail. Another advantage is that it allows for ventilation and oxygenation during two steps in the process, which is of benefit if the fiberoptic process is difficult and takes more time than usual. Finally, with some experience, the whole procedure takes no more than 5 min, and is virtually 100 % reliable.

An alternative Plan C involves using the Aintree catheter as the guide for inserting the endotracheal tube (Video 4.9). The Aintree catheter is a 56 cm long hollow tube that will slide over a standard fiberoptic bronchoscope. Using an LMA or airway as a guide, the fiberoptic scope is inserted into the trachea and the Aintree catheter is slid into the trachea. The scope and LMA or airway are removed and an endotracheal tube is inserted over the Aintree catheter into the trachea. The advantage of the Aintree catheter is that as soon as it is in place, the endotracheal tube can be inserted. The disadvantages of the Aintree catheter are twofold. First, one must be facile with the fiberoptic bronchoscope because all of the scope control and movements must be done from the scope handle. One cannot make small adjustments in the scope position by manipulating the shaft of the scope because the Aintree catheter fits loosely around the scope shaft preventing any more distal movement of the scope using the shaft. Second, one must work quickly as there is no opportunity to ventilate the lungs from the start of the intubation until its completion. If the fiberoptic procedure itself proves to be difficult, the patient may become desaturated before the intubation can be completed.

Plan D (Video 4.10)

If Plans A–C fail, one needs Plan D. The first and perhaps the most prudent option is to cancel the proposed operation, terminate the anesthetic, reverse the neuromuscular blockade, and wake the patient up. The operation would be rescheduled for another day, and at that time an awake fiberoptic intubation technique would be used. Alternatively, if the operation cannot be postponed, then the surgeon should be informed that a surgical airway (i.e.: tracheostomy) must be performed before the planned operation can commence. To date, utilization of Plan D because of failure of Plans A–C has not occurred.

Other Devices

There are many other devices currently available for assisting with a difficult intubation (Video 4.11). Perhaps one of the most useful among them is the Intubating LMA (Video 4.12). This device has many advocates and has been used successfully in both elective and emergency circumstances. When it works, it can be a lifesaving device. Its major drawback is that in difficult intubations it may not always work, even with multiple attempts by experienced operators. Another device is the Air-Q LMA, which has been advocated for use in difficult intubations (Video 4.13). Its limitations are that the largest tube that can be easily inserted through it is a 6.5 OD, and success with its use in a broad variety of difficult intubations is not documented.

There is very little place in the management of the difficult airway for such devices as the light wand, the Bullard or other specialized laryngoscopes, or the implementation of transtracheal jet ventilation. All of these techniques have a low degree of reliability in the hands of the average anesthesiologist, and consume valuable time when an urgent of emergency airway is needed. Retrograde intubation is a useful, **elective technique** for patients with markedly distorted airways. It involves insertion of a needle into the cricothyroid membrane, threading of a guide wire through the needle cephalad until it can be grasped in the back of the mouth, threading a small airway exchange catheter (AEC) down the guide wire, and then inserting a small endotracheal tube over the AEC. The guide wire and AEC can then be pulled out through the mouth.

Cervical Spine Injury

There are three basic approaches to accomplishing endotracheal intubation in patients with confirmed or suspected cervical spine injury. They are: awake fiberoptic intubation; asleep either with direct or fiberoptic laryngoscopy and using in-line traction (Gardner-Wells tongs) or manual stabilization; and Plan C. One or other of the first two techniques has been the standard management for many years and continues to the present. However, both of the first two techniques have serious flaws.

The awake fiberoptic technique necessitates prior topicalization of the oropharynx and trachea, which to be effective will precipitate coughing of unknown magnitude and duration. Either vigorous coughing or bucking during topicalization or insertion of the tube may injure the spinal cord further. Also, satisfactory topicalization may be virtually impossible to accomplish in patients with a smoking history or a strong gag reflex.

If intubation is performed under anesthesia using in-line traction or manual stabilization, there is no assurance that either method will adequately protect the spinal cord during the head manipulation that is often required with direct laryngoscopy. In fact, a recent study found that manual in-line stabilization worsened glottis visualization with a Macintosh #3 blade, and that pressures applied to the oropharyngeal tissues were substantially greater than without its use [2]. The investigators concluded that manual in-line stabilization and standard laryngoscopy have the potential for causing distortion of the craniocervical axis. Using a videolaryngoscope such as the GlideScope® is no safer since it has been shown that although the visualization is improved, the craniocervical motion is as severe as with the Macintosh blade [3]. Another group has advocated the use of the Airtraq video laryngoscope for endotracheal intubation of patients with cervical spine immobilization. While its performance was better than the Macintosh blade, neck movement of unknown severity occurred even though anesthesiologists experienced in the use of this blade performed the intubations [4].

In contrast, Plan C is the best first choice technique for intubation of the trachea in patients with possible or known cervical spine fracture or injury. Plan C is ideal because it does not involve any movement of the head or neck to establish endotracheal intubation. Most of these patients will come to the operating room in a cervical collar or occasionally a Halo jacket, both of which can be left in place during intubation. If there is concern about aspiration during induction, cricoid pressure can be used during Plan C until the trachea is secured. The only caveat to using Plan C as the plan of choice in these or any patients is the need to confirm that bag-mask ventilation or ventilation with an LMA is possible under light anesthesia before moving forward. This is because Plan C is always performed with patients anesthetized and paralyzed.

Extubation Strategy

Having an extubation strategy is just as important as having an intubation strategy when dealing with patients who have a difficult airway. Included in the extubation strategy are the usual concerns that the patients be awake, conscious and responsive, have full neuromuscular function, and can maintain normal oxygen and carbon dioxide levels while breathing spontaneously. While waiting for full emergence it may be helpful to spray lidocaine down the endotracheal tube using a laryngotracheal anesthesia (LTA) kit to minimize coughing during emergence. At this point, if there is any concern about the patient's ability to maintain an airway after extubation, two options are available. One is to sedate the patient either with spontaneous or controlled ventilation and leave the endotracheal tube in overnight, and reassess the patient's condition the next day. The other option is to occlude the endotracheal tube at its connector and with the pilot balloon down determine if the patient is able to breathe around the tube. Either with or without that test, the anesthesiologist can insert an AEC below the level of the endotracheal tube and remove the tube. If the AEC does not touch the carina and it is not moved, the patient will tolerate it without coughing and it can be removed some time later. The AEC will not significantly affect the patient's ability to speak. If the patient should develop respiratory distress or failure after extubation, the AEC will act as an ideal conduit for reintroducing an endotracheal tube.

When is Tracheal Intubation Not Indicated for Respiratory Failure?

The mantra of anesthesia is to intubate the trachea whenever possible for the treatment of severe respiratory distress or respiratory failure. However, one circumstance where intubation is **not indicated** is a patient with respiratory distress from an enlarging hematoma in the neck. This may occur following a variety of surgical procedures including thyroidectomy, parotidectomy, carotid endarterectomy or isolation of carotid vessels for control of bleeding during ligation of an intracranial aneurysm. When this occurs, the patient usually complains of difficulty breathing. On examination, the airway is generally so deviated and distorted by the hematoma that intubation is impossible, and attempted intubation results in worsening of the respiratory status and wastes valuable time. The immediate treatment is evacuation of the hematoma, compression of the neck to minimize further bleeding, and return of the patient to the operating room where intubation can be accomplished under controlled conditions.

Fiberoptic Intubation of the Trachea

When planning fiberoptic intubation (FOL) two decisions must be made at the out-set: namely, oral vs. nasal approach, which is usually a surgical decision, and awake vs. asleep. Generally the asleep FOL is easier and quicker for both patients and the anesthesiologist, especially in those patients with a strong gag reflex or those who have been longstanding smokers. Achieving adequate topical anesthesia in these groups of patients is challenging and often unsatisfactory. Sedation for awake FOL can be accomplished using midazolam, fentanyl, or a continuous infusion of propo-fol or dexmedetomidine (Video 4.14). Topicalization of the oropharynx is best accomplished using lidocaine 4 % aerosolized using an atomizer, asking the patient to breathe deeply during spraying. One can check for loss of the gag reflex by apply-ing lidocaine jelly 2 % on a tongue depressor and inserting it the back of the orophar-ynx. Once the gag reflex is abolished, it is advisable to do a transtracheal injection of local anesthetic, preferably cocaine 4%. Although it may cause some coughing, doing a transtracheal injection has two benefits: one, it provides topical anesthesia below the level of the vocal cords, lessening the chance for severe coughing when the fiberoptic scope and endotracheal tube are inserted; and two, it gives the operator experience identifying the thyroid and cricoid cartilages and inserting a needle through the cricothyroid membrane. The knowledge and experience obtained by doing multiple transtracheal injections are invaluable for overcoming reluctance and increasing the success rate if called upon to perform an emergency cricothyrotomy (Video 4.15). Cocaine 4 % (up to 3 mg/kg) is the best drug for transtracheal injection because it works faster and produces a more profound block than any other local anesthetic; and because it produces local vasoconstriction which limits any bleeding at the block site. It is advisable to have patients breathing oxygen before performing the transtracheal injection, because a small fraction of patients will develop laryngo-spasm following the injection. However, the laryngospasm will resolve spontane-ously very quickly because to the local effect of the cocaine.

Once topical anesthesia is complete, the fiberoptic scope is mounted with an endotracheal tube (a 7.0 OD is large enough for any adult, and the smaller the tube, the easier the advancement into the trachea), and inserted through an oral guide, either a Tudor-Williams (T-W), Patel or Ovassapian airway. Each of the airways has its advantages. The T-W airway has a distinctive pink color that makes identifying it from patient tissues easy, while the other airways are white and less distinguishable from oropharyngeal tissues. Removal of the T-W airway from the mouth once the endotracheal tube is in position is more difficult owing to the need to remove the tube adaptor from the tube in order to remove the airway from the mouth. In contrast, the other two airways can be removed with the tube connector in place. It is advisable to lubricate the endotracheal tube before advancing it into the trachea. If it does not advance easily, the tube should be rotated slightly counterclockwise to bring its tip closer to the midline of the tracheal opening. The operator must be very gentle advancing the tube to avoid any injury to the vocal cords. Sometimes multiple, gentle attempts at advancement need to be made before the tube enters the trachea. Because tube insertion is blind, it is necessary to confirm its location as endotracheal and not endobronchial by balloting the pilot balloon with a syringe and palpating the bounce at or above the sternal notch.

If the nasal route is desired, it is necessary to topicalize the nasal cavity (Video 4.16). Again, the best choice is cocaine 4% soaked in cotton applicators that can be gently introduced into the nasal cavity. The vasoconstrictor effect of cocaine (by preventing the reuptake of norepinephrine) offers the best chance for minimizing nasal bleeding from insertion of the applicators. After inserting several applicators, it is advisable to introduce graduated nasal dilators up to the size of the nasotracheal tube to be used. For most patients, a 6.0–7.0 OD nasal RAE tube is optimal. As the fiberoptic scope is introduced into the nose, the operator should ask an assistant to provide forward displacement of the mandible to open up the oropharynx. With the scope in the midline and slightly flexed, it will generally be easy to advance the scope into the trachea. It is important to have the scope well into the trachea **before** advancing the nasotracheal tube through the nasal cavity so that any bleeding from the nasotracheal tube advancement does not obscure visualization of the glottis opening.

Videolaryngoscopy

One of the significant advances in airway management has been the development of videolaryngoscopy. The basic technique involved the use of a camera attached to an airway device such as a laryngoscope, with the view or picture being transmitted to a screen for visualization by the operator. A number of devices have been developed, the most popular being the GlideScope®, because of is adaptability, ease of use, and image quality. The GlideScope® (Fig. 4.3) consists of a single use or reusable Macintosh blade (sizes 3–5) attached to a cord, which provides a bright light at the tip of the blade and which transmits the view to the screen, which is on a portable, moveable stand. With the operating room lights dimmed, the picture is a clear, color image of the anatomical view (Fig. 4.4). A rigid stylet is inserted into the endotracheal tube that is to be used, which conforms the tube to the same curvature as the blade. Once the tube is at the laryngeal opening, the stylet is retracted a few centimeters using the bar attached to the distal portion of the stylet, and the tube is advanced into the laryngeal opening. As the tube with stylet is advanced into the oropharynx, it is essential for the operator to watch its advancement in the mouth, not on the screen. Failure to do so may result in inadvertent perforation of soft tissue in the oropharynx. This error may result in an oropharyngeal abscess, an oropharyngeal fistula and mediastinal abscess, and/or mediastinal emphysema. One author [5] has suggested that videolaryngoscopy should be used routinely and be the new standard of care. We would argue that for an anesthesiologist the maintenance of alternative airway management skills requires continuous practice that could not be achieved with over-reliance on video laryngoscopy.

Fig. 4.3 GlideScope on portable stand. Courtesy of Verathon Medical

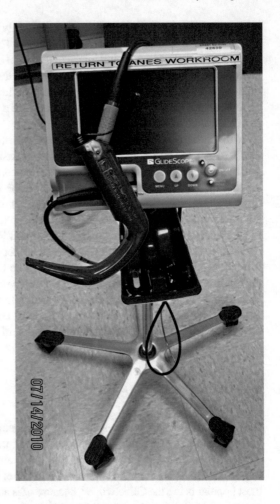

As useful as the GlideScope® and other video laryngoscopes are, it must be acknowledged that they are not a perfect solution to airway management, because they do not always provide a view that will permit tracheal intubation. Plan C will still be necessary to accomplish tracheal intubation when attempts with video laryngoscopes fail.

Tying the Tracheal Tube (Video 4.17)

Once the breathing tube is properly positioned in the trachea, it is mandatory that it be fixed at that location so that it neither migrates inward causing an endobronchial intubation and one lung ventilation, nor migrates outward resulting in loss of the airway. Generally, tracheal tubes are secured with tape, but there are circumstances

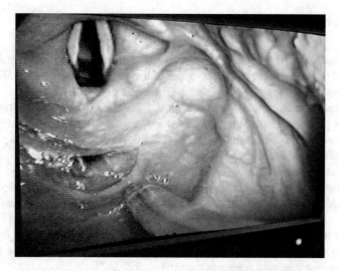

Fig. 4.4 View of laryngeal opening with GlideScope blade inserted in oropharynx. Courtesy of Verathon Medical

where tape is unreliable. For example, it is often impossible to secure the tube with tape in men with heavy beards and mustache. Some patients have paper-like facial skin that has the potential for peeling away from the face as the tape is removed. Some patients have extremely oily skin to which tape will not adhere even after prepping the facial skin with an adhesive-like liquid. In such circumstances it is best to secure the tube position by tying it to the neck or by wiring the tube to the teeth.

There are several ways to obtain cervical fixation, but one of the easiest is to tie a tight knot on the tube at the level of the lips using umbilical tape. One end of the tape should be long enough to pass behind the patient's neck and then tied to the other end of the tape in a bow at the side of the neck. Once tied, there should be no slack in the tape, but it should not be so tight that it effects the venous drainage from the head and neck. Once completed, pulling gently on the tube should not result in any appreciable movement. Using a bow knot makes it easy to untie the tape when it is time for removal of the tube.

Interdental wire fixation of the endotracheal tube is a useful alternative when circumferential neck fixation must be avoided. In this method a length of fine dental wire is passed through the interdental space lateral to one of the upper incisors, looped behind both upper incisors and back out through the opposite interdental space. The wire is then secured to the two upper incisors by twisting the wires together using a needle holder. After about ten twists, the free ends of the wires are twice wrapped around the endotracheal tube and twisted together until the wire indents the endotracheal tube. Proper fixation of the endotracheal tube should be tested, and the excess wire is trimmed and coiled to prevent the sharp ends from traumatizing adjacent tissue. Extubation is accomplished after the incisor loop is cut using wire cutters. The wire can then be removed from between the teeth and the endotracheal tube removed with all of the wire still attached.

Insertion of Double-Lumen Tubes (Video 4.18)

It has been standard practice for many years to insert a double-lumen tube in the trachea of patients undergoing many types of lung surgery. This practice allowed for deflation of one lung while maintaining ventilation of the other lung. Until recently, the left endobronchial tube was used almost exclusively because the right endo-bronchial tube was much more difficult to insert safely. When positioning the right endobronchial it is critical that the most proximal orifice on the tube be positioned over the takeoff of the bronchus to the right upper lobed to ensure ventilation of that lobe. With the advent of fiberoptic scopes, it is much easier to visualize the bron-chial structures and position with great accuracy both left or right endobronchial tubes. While thoracic auscultation is still used, direct visualization through each endobronchial lumen using a fiberoptic scope has become the standard of practice. Since the tube position can change with changes in patient positioning (i.e.: supine to lateral), it is necessary to check endobronchial tube location with the fiberoptic scope once the final positioning is completed.

Endobronchial blockers can be an effective and simple alternative to the use of double-lumen endotracheal tubes. The EZ-Blocker™ endobronchial blocker is a substantial improvement over conventional endobronchial blockers. As shown in Fig. 4.5, it has a bifurcated end with two inflatable cuffs designed to be deployed across the carina following insertion though a standard 7.0 or larger endotracheal tube using the supplied adapter. The tip of the endotracheal tube must be at least 4 cm above the carina to permit proper deployment of the bifurcated tips. The EZ-Blocker™ is inserted through the adapter along with a flexible bronchoscope. Under direct observation, the blocker is advanced until the two ends are in the

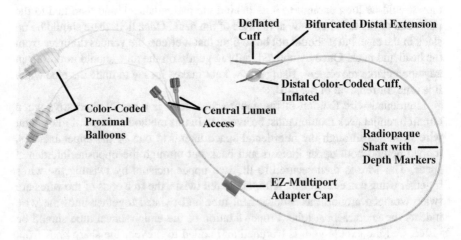

Fig. 4.5 EZ-Blocker™ endobronchial blocker with individual components identified. Its bifur-cated tip design makes correct placement relatively simple. Courtesy of Teleflex Medical Incorporated

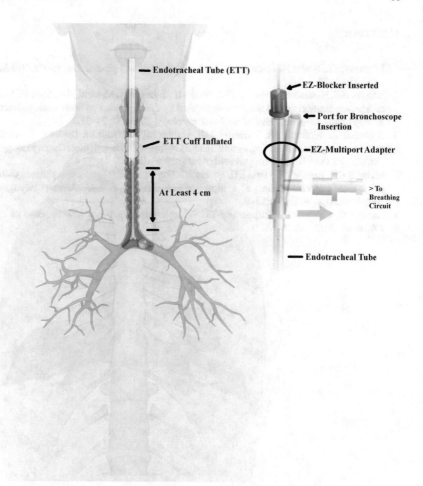

Fig. 4.6 Following intubation the EZ-Multiport Adapter is attached and proper ETT placement with the tip at least 4 cm above the carina is verified. The EZ-Blocker™ is inserted until the bifurcated ends are in each bronchus. Blocker placement and orientation are confirmed by inflating and deflating the cuffs under direct bronchoscopic observation. As shown in the figure, the cuff in the left main bronchus has been inflated to isolate the left lung, permitting unimpeded ventilation of the right lung. Courtesy of Teleflex Medical Incorporated

mainstem bronchi, and orientation is verified by inflating and deflating each cuff. Ventilation is suspended until lung collapse is achieved. The cuff in the bronchus of the lung to be isolated is then inflated and ventilation resumed (Fig. 4.6). [The manufacturer should be contacted for complete instructions including precautions and warnings before use.]

Acknowledgement Video credits in Video 4.19.

References

1. Magnusson L, Spahn DR. New concepts of atelectasis during general anaesthesia. Br J Anaesth. 2003;91:61–72.
2. Santoni BG, Hindman BJ, Puttlitz CM, Weeks JB, Johnson N, Maktabi MA, Todd MM. Manual in-line stabilization increases pressures applied by the laryngoscope blade during direct laryngoscopy and orotracheal intubation. Anesthesiology. 2009;110:24–31.
3. Robitaille A, Williams SR, Tremblay MH, Guilbert F, Theriault M, Drolet P. Cervical spine motion during tracheal intubation with manual in-line stabilization: direct laryngoscopy versus GlideScope videolaryngoscopy. Anesth Analg. 2008;106:935–41.
4. Maharaj CH, Buckley E, Harte BH, Laffey JG. Endotracheal intubation in patients with cervical spine immobilization: a comparison of Macintosh and Airtraq laryngoscopes. Anesthesiology. 2007;107:53–9.
5. Zaouter C, Calderon J, Hemmerling TM. Videolaryngoscopy as a new standard of care. Br J Anaesth. 2015;114:181–3.

Chapter 5
Laryngospasm: The Silent Menace

Introduction

Laryngospasm is defined as the involuntary spasm or contraction of the muscles of the larynx resulting in total occlusion of the airway. It occurs most commonly during emergence from general anesthesia, usually immediately after removal of a tracheal tube, laryngeal mask airway, or other airway device. Rarely, it may also occur in unanaesthetized subjects should they be at risk for pulmonary aspiration from, for example, gastroesophageal reflux disease. The reason that "silent" is in the title of this chapter is because laryngospasm does not create any sound. Laryngeal stridor is accompanied by a high-pitched, striderous sound of varying intensity as gas transgresses the glottic opening. In contrast, laryngospasm is totally noiseless because no gas passes the tightly closed glottis. The deceiving part is that the chest appears to be moving in a regular manner, suggesting ventilation. However, the experienced eye immediately recognizes that the pattern of movement of the chest is quite abnormal. Instead of rising normally with inhalation, the upper chest and suprasternal neck collapse inward in response to the negative intrathoracic pressure generated by the inspiratory effort. At the same time, the lower chest and abdomen may move downward and outward, again suggesting that ventilation is occurring, which it is not.

> **Signs of Laryngospasm**
> - Absence of ventilatory sounds
> - Inward movement of upper chest with inhalation
> - Downward, outward movement of lower chest and abdomen with inhalation
> - Inability to ventilate the lungs with bag-mask

Electronic supplementary material: The online version of this chapter (doi:10.1007/978-3-319-42866-6_5) contains supplementary material, which is available to authorized users. Videos can also be accessed at http://link.springer.com/chapter/10.1007/978-3-319-42866-6_5.

© Springer International Publishing Switzerland 2017
C.P. Larson Jr., R.A. Jaffe, *Practical Anesthetic Management*,
DOI 10.1007/978-3-319-42866-6_5

- Deteriorating oxygen saturation despite oxygen administration by mask
- Presence of pink-tinged fluid in the oropharynx

Although the Chest and Abdomen are Moving, There are No Breath Sounds When Laryngospasm is Present

The reason that the word "menace" is used in the title of this chapter is because laryngospasm can cause serious complications and even death. Three actual cases are cited as examples of what can happen when laryngospasm is not promptly diagnosed and treated.

Case 1

A 22 year old, otherwise healthy man was admitted to hospital for removal of nasal polyps under general anesthesia. After placement of standard monitors, anesthesia was induced with fentanyl, propofol, and succinylcholine, and an endotracheal tube was inserted. Anesthesia was maintained with sevoflurane–oxygen. At the conclusion of the 55-min operation, spontaneous ventilation was established and the sevoflurane was discontinued. Soon thereafter, he responded to commands to take a deep breath and the endotracheal tube was removed. A mask from the anesthesia circuit was placed on his face with an oxygen flow of 8 L/min. He appeared to be breathing adequately, but after a few minutes, the oxygen saturation began to decline below 90 %. Positive pressure ventilation via mask with jaw thrust was attempted without success. The patient was given succinylcholine 60 mg i/v, and after 2–3 min positive pressure ventilation was established. Shortly thereafter, pink-stained fluid began to come out of his mouth. His airway was suctioned; he was placed on a CPAP mask with 100 % oxygen; put in a semi-sitting position; and given a single dose of furosemide. Over the next 12 h, his oxygen saturation, which was in the mid-80s gradually increased to the mid-90s. He was admitted to hospital and discharged on the second postoperative day with a normal saturation breathing room air. *The finding of pink-tinged fluid in the oropharynx several minutes after extubation of the trachea suggests that laryngospasm may have caused negative pressure pulmonary edema.*

Case 2

A 72 year old, 188-pound man was admitted to hospital for radiation treatment for cancer of the prostate. His other medical problems were hypertension and non-insulin dependent diabetes. His vital signs and laboratory values were within normal limits and he was rated an ASA II. The surgical plan was to place radiation seeds into the prostate, and the anesthetic plan was general anesthesia with insertion of an LMA. Anesthesia was induced with midazolam, fentanyl, propofol, and low dose rocuronium. An LMA #4 was inserted and anesthesia was maintained with desflurane–oxygen.

Controlled ventilation was instituted and the patient was placed in lithotomy position. Shortly thereafter, peak airway pressure, which had been below 20 cmH$_2$O, rapidly increased to greater than 30 cmH$_2$O. The LMA was repositioned without improvement, so it was removed and replaced. Ventilation still could not be established so the LMA was removed and bag-mask ventilation attempted after insertion of an oral airway. This was also unsuccessful. Direct laryngoscopy was attempted but only the tip of the epiglottis could be visualized. Multiple subsequent attempts at intubation using a blind technique, the Fastrach LMA™, and fiberoptic intubation were unsuccessful. The patient went into cardiac arrest and cardiopulmonary resuscitation was started. Ultimately, a #6 endotracheal tube was passed under direct laryngoscopy, but the patient died several days later. The cause of death was deemed to be prolonged hypoxemia secondary to mechanical obstruction of the airway from laryngospasm and subsequent inability to ventilate the lungs or intubate the trachea.

Case 3

This case is that of Joan Rivers, the famous comedienne who had an untoward event in an outpatient facility in New York City. The facts cited here are those widely circulated in the press and on television following the event. Ms. Rivers went into an outpatient facility for an esophagoscopy under intravenous sedation because of a history of gastroesophageal reflux. During the esophagoscopy, a lesion was noted on a vocal cord, and an ear, nose and throat specialist was consulted. A biopsy of the lesion was performed, and immediately thereafter Ms. Rivers went into complete airway obstruction. Attempts to reestablish ventilation failed and she went into cardiopulmonary arrest. Ultimately an airway and circulation were established, but she did not regain consciousness and died about a week later in a nearby hospital.

Case Discussion

Case 1 is an example of the most common, serious complication of undiagnosed and untreated laryngospasm, namely negative pressure pulmonary edema (NPPE). NPPE can occur in any age group, but is most common in young healthy men, probably because of the high negative intrathoracic pressure that they can generate with their strong thoracic and abdominal musculature. The appearance of normal ventilation was deceptive and delayed establishing effective treatment. He made a full recovery but not before a period of considerable anguish by the patient, his family, and the physicians and nurses caring for him.

Case 2 is an example of the most deleterious outcome from undetected laryngospasm and subsequent inability to ventilate the lungs or intubate the trachea. This case demonstrates three points: (1) attempts at ventilation with an LMA or bag and mask may not be successful in resolving laryngospasm regardless of the airway pressure applied; (2) attempts at tracheal intubation are futile as it is impossible to identify the laryngeal opening or insert a tube into the trachea when the vocal cords are in spasm; and (3) use of other airway devices such as a fiberoptic scope are not likely to be successful.

Case 3 is a classic scenario in which acute laryngospasm will occur. The combination of sedation or light anesthesia (not general anesthesia) and irritation of the vocal cords, in this case by a biopsy of a lesion on a vocal cord caused the laryngospasm. While uncommon, the sequence of events in Cases 2 and 3 are not what might be called exceedingly rare. Lack of space, not lack of material, prevents citation of other cases of death following laryngospasm. What is rare is that these cases are seldom, if ever, reported in the literature, and hence their true incidence is unknown. This case, because of the international fame of the patient, does draw attention to the problem of laryngospasm. What these cases do show is that positive pressure ventilation, as a primary therapy, may be ineffective.

Functional Anatomy of the Larynx

B. Raymond Fink published two classic texts on the functional anatomy of the human larynx [1, 2]. His interest in this subject emanated from his clinical experiences with laryngospasm at the conclusion of general anesthesia. What his detailed analysis showed was that closure of the glottic opening during laryngospasm is not a simple matter, but involves a complex set of movements in the larynx (Fig. 5.1).

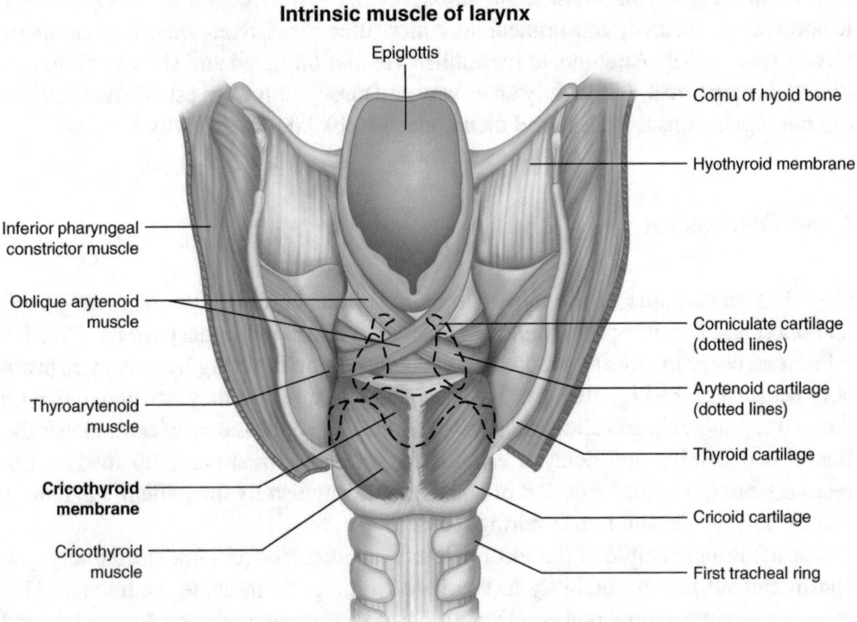

Fig. 5.1 Schematic illustration of the structures of the larynx including the muscles and most importantly the cricothyroid membrane where the cricothyrotomy is performed

This would include contracture of the muscles of the laryngeal inlet (oblique arytenoid and aryepiglottic muscles), the adductors of the glottis (lateral cricoarytenoid and transverse arytenoid muscles), the tensors of the vocal cords (cricothyroid muscles), and the abductor of the vocal folds (posterior cricoarytenoid muscles). In addition, Fink and his colleague, R. J. Demarest postulated that the human larynx is a system of articulating cartilages suspended by muscles and ligaments from the hyoid bone, mandible and even the base of the skull. This allows the larynx to undergo "respiratory folding or bellows folding" during exhalation and unfolding during inhalation. This folding phenomenon would further narrow the laryngeal opening during laryngospasm. Thus it is no surprise that when one views by direct laryngoscopy the larynx in spasm, all one sees is a mass of tissue where the laryngeal opening should be.

Prevention of Laryngospasm

Over the years there have been a number of techniques devised for preventing laryngospasm at the conclusion of anesthesia and extubation of the trachea. The most effective of these is extubation of the trachea while the patient is still in surgical anesthesia, since laryngospasm will not occur at this level of anesthesia. However, there are several downsides to this technique. First, a patent airway must be maintained until the patient emerges from general anesthesia. This may not be easy or safe in some patients for a variety of reasons. Second, the technique cannot be used in patients with a history of a full stomach. And third, there is no guarantee that laryngospasm will not occur anyway during emergence. The combination of light anesthesia and irritation of the larynx by secretions may precipitate laryngospasm even though the trachea was extubated early. Other techniques include avoidance of drugs such as desflurane that might have a penchant for causing laryngospasm, or spraying the trachea with lidocaine before or the larynx immediately after extubation of the trachea. The effectiveness of these techniques has not been established. *The conclusion is that* there is no guaranteed technique for preventing laryngospasm.

Treatment of Laryngospasm

Just as with prevention, there have been a number of treatment options offered over the years for treating laryngospasm. The most commonly recommended technique is positive pressure ventilation with bag and mask, with or without simultaneous jaw thrust. Jaw thrust, or forward displacement of the mandible is generally performed at the angle of the jaw. While this maneuver will correct airway obstruction from the tongue, because as the jaw moves forward the tongue comes forward owing to traction on the genioglossus muscle, which is attached between the tongue and mandible, it will not correct laryngospasm. Positive pressure ventilation is ineffective against a closed glottis until the patient becomes sufficiently hypoxemic that the vocal cords and laryngeal muscles relax. To overcome this problem it is usually recommended that the patient be given a small dose of succinylcholine (0.5 mg/kg) i/v or a somewhat larger dose intramuscularly. However, administering succinylcholine, even in small doses, is both unnecessary and potentially dangerous. The muscle fasciculations, the release of potassium into the blood, and the arrhythmias that may occur are all potentially life threatening. Also, since one cannot predict when laryngospasm may occur on emergence, this solution means that every anesthesia provider must have a syringe of succinylcholine immediately available for administration during every general anesthetic. On a national scale, this represents substantial additional cost of anesthesia and tremendous waste of drug when it is not used. It is of interest to note that there is no scientific study documenting either the efficacy or reliability of jaw thrust and positive pressure ventilation for treating laryngospasm. Obviously, positive pressure ventilation is not reliable or there would be no need to administer succinylcholine as part of the technique.

Larson described the best treatment of laryngospasm in an article in 1998 [3–4] (Video 5.1). The technique involves identifying what has been named the laryngospasm notch. This bony notch is just behind the ear lobe and is bounded anteriorly by the coronoid process of the mandible, posteriorly by the mastoid process, and superiorly by the base of the skull (Fig. 5.2). With the patient lying supine, a finger is placed in the notch on each side of the head and very firm pressure is directed straight inward while at the same time pulling upward (skyward) on the coronoid process. Properly performed, the laryngospasm should resolve within 15–30 s. The technique simultaneously corrects airway obstruction from the tongue as well as from laryngospasm owing to the forward displacement of the mandible by the maneuver. The two most important steps in the laryngospasm maneuver are: (1) making certain that the operator can *feel the base of the skull*; and (2) pushing inward and upward in a *very firm* manner. (A video of the technique being performed on a manikin is attached here, and a video of it being performed on a patient is available from the New England Journal of Medicine, (N Engl J Med 2014, 370:1266–68). The technique works equally well in infants, children and adults. Generally the technique is applied to both laryngospasm notches, but it works even if only one notch is available because of head or neck surgery. The technique should be performed *routinely* immediately after extubation of the trachea since one cannot tell for a while by looking at patients whether they are in laryngospasm or not. It is advisable to place a transport mask delivering oxygen on the patient's face while doing the maneuver. Using the oxygen mask from the anesthesia circuit is not recommended because it is hard to hold the mask in place while doing the maneuver. The technique should be continued until the patient is able to reach up and attempt to stop the pressure. This response by the patient has been named the Larson reflex. Once this occurs, it is exceedingly rare that a patient will go back into laryngospasm. By doing this maneuver automatically after every tracheal extubation, anesthesia providers become very proficient in its application and come to realize that the concern for and complications of laryngospasm are a thing of the past (Fig. 5.3).

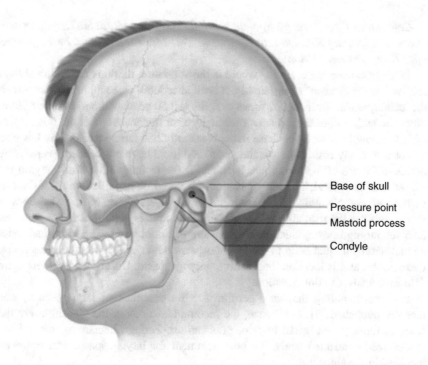

Fig. 5.2 Schematic illustration of laryngospasm notch bounded anteriorly by the coronoid process of the mandible (labeled condyle), posteriorly by the mastoid process, and superiorly by the base of the skull. Digital pressure is applied firmly directly inward and upward on each side of the head at the apex of the notch as shown by the *red* dot. The pressure point is behind the most cephalad portion of the ear lobe where it joins the cartilage of the ear (not shown)

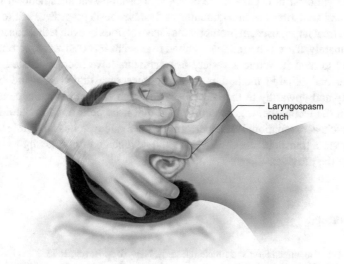

Fig. 5.3 Example of the application of pressure at the laryngospasm notch to prevent or treat laryngospasm

Continuous Firm Pressure Applied Inwardly and Upwardly at the Laryngospasm Notch will Quickly Resolve Laryngospasm. This Maneuver should be Performed after Every Tracheal Extubation.

Three questions arise. First, "where is the validation that this technique always resolves laryngospasm"? Regrettably, it is all anecdotal. One author has performed the technique well over 20,000 times over the last 50 years without a single failure. Since the author does the maneuver routinely after tracheal extubation, it is impossible to know how many of these patients actually had laryngospasm. He has also taught it to many residents over the years, and there have not been any reports by others of failure of the technique. Second, "is the technique harmful"? Again the evidence is anecdotal. The author has not observed or identified any transient or permanent complications from performing the maneuver. Third, "why does it work...what is the mechanism"? While the technique is painful, it is not pain that resolves laryngospasm, since pain elsewhere does not work. The ninth and tenth cranial nerves lie just deep to the laryngospasm notch, and it may be pressure on these nerves at this location that resolves laryngospasm. Unfortunately, there is no definitive answer to this question.

It is worth noting that an algorithm for the treatment of laryngospasm was recently published [5]. In essence, the recommendations in the algorithm are the same as those promulgated in prior publications. Perhaps because of the lack of randomized controlled trials, the best treatment for laryngospasm was not even included in the algorithm.

Summary

When laryngospasm occurs at the conclusion of a general anesthetic, it is disconcerting and sometimes even frightening to the anesthesia provider. Failure to recognize and treat laryngospasm promptly may have serious or even lethal consequences. Unfortunately, there is no reliable method to prevent its occurrence, so one must be prepared to treat it. While a variety of treatments have been suggested, the most effective and reliable method is to apply very firm digital pressure bilaterally inwardly and upwardly at the laryngospasm notch. To gain experience and confidence in the technique, it is recommended that it be performed immediately after every tracheal extubation. While performing the maneuver, it is advisable to provide oxygen via a transport mask, which has the advantage of not having to be held in place by the provider.

References

1. Fink BR. The human larynx: a functional study. New York: Raven; 1975.
2. Fink BR, Demarest RJ. Laryngeal biomechanics. Cambridge, MA: Harvard University Press; 1978.

3. Larson CP. Laryngospasm, the best treatment. Anesthesiology. 1998;89:1293.
4. Larson CP. Laryngospasm: a continuing problem. In: Morgan Jr GE, Mikhail MS, Murray MJ, editors. Clinical anesthesiology. 3rd ed. New York: Lange Medical Books; 2002. p. 78–9.
5. Ramez Salem M, Crystal GJ, Nimmagadda U. Understanding the mechanism of laryngospasm is crucial for proper treatment. Anesthesiology. 2012;117:441–2.

Chapter 6
Cricothyrotomy: A Lesson to Be Learned

Unfortunately on rare occasions, anesthesia providers will experience patients whose lungs cannot be ventilated using a bag-mask technique, an LMA or a tracheal tube. When this occurs, the only alternative may be to do an emergency cricothyrotomy. In this circumstance the central issue is: "Should one use a knife or a needle to establish an emergency airway?" The only reason that there is any debate about this matter is that most anesthesia personnel have no real life experience with either technique, and hence have no way to judge which is better. However, in a life-threatening airway obstruction, there is no question which is better. An emergency cricothyrotomy using a knife is much quicker, easier, safer and more effective than any needle-based technique. There should be no place in emergency airway management for needle-based attempts to establish ventilation. It should be deleted from the ASA Difficult Airway Algorithm, but it probably won't be because many of the members who design or evaluate the algorithm have never performed either technique in an emergency. The authors have participated in nine cricothyrotomies in emergency airway situations, and all the patients left the hospital without any neurological injury or complications from the cricothyrotomy. Although there are no randomized controlled trials, we believe that the risk-benefit ratio markedly favors the knife technique.

First, a knife cricothyrotomy is quicker and easier since one can find the cricothyroid membrane or tracheal rings and trachea much faster with a knife or scissors than with a needle. We have been teaching routine transtracheal injections to residents for over 50 years, and even after multiple attempts experienced residents still struggle to find the cricothyroid membrane. In an emergency, that delay is unacceptable. With a knife or scissors one cuts quickly either vertically or horizontally through the skin of the neck and then through the cricothyroid membrane, which lies between the thyroid cartilage above and the cricoid cartilage below. The knife is inserted into the trachea and turned 90°, and an airway is established (Fig. 6.1). At that point a small tube of any type can be inserted next to the knife. The knife technique is much safer because there is virtually nothing that one can harm by

© Springer International Publishing Switzerland 2017
C.P. Larson Jr., R.A. Jaffe, *Practical Anesthetic Management*,
DOI 10.1007/978-3-319-42866-6_6

Fig. 6.1 Midline incision
at the level of the junction
between the thyroid and
cricoid cartilages
(cricothyroid membrane).
Permission for use granted
by Cook Medical,
Bloomington, Indiana

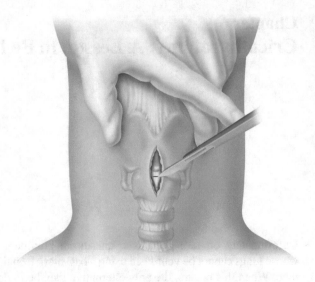

making an incision near the midline of the neck, and it can be performed in less than 30 s. In contrast, the needle technique is fraught with major problems. These include: identifying the trachea; making certain that the needle is entirely in the trachea, and does not move to avoid causing massive subcutaneous emphysema when an oxygen source is established; establishing a pressurized oxygen delivery system, which will take more than 5 min even in the most experienced environment; and avoiding causing a tension pneumothorax with ventilation against a closed glottis. Finally, the knife technique is more effective. We know of multiple cases of acute airway obstruction where the needle technique was attempted, and in all cases the patient died. We know of no such cases where a knife cricothyrotomy was used as the primary treatment of unresolved acute airway obstruction.

In a recently, nationally publicized case, an internist successfully performed a knife cricothyrotomy in a restaurant following a failed Mueller maneuver in an overweight woman who developed acute airway obstruction from a piece of meat. If an internist can do this in a restaurant, anesthesia providers should be able to do it in the more controlled setting of an operating room or hospital. DITCH THE NEEDLE AND USE THE KNIFE!

Recently, the national press focused attention on a young girl on life support at Children's Hospital, Oakland. At issue was a dispute between hospital officials who wanted to terminate ventilator care and the mother who refused such action, even though expert neurologists uniformly confirmed that the girl was clinically brain dead. We do not intend to discuss the pros and cons of that issue, but rather to consider what caused the brain death in the first place. The specific facts of the case are not known, and because of litigation probably will not be for many years, if ever. However it is not difficult from public information to surmise the essence of what might have happened, and thereby construct a lesson to be learned.

The girl had chronic, recurrent, partial obstructive airway disease as a result of enlarged tonsils and adenoids in combination with childhood obesity. Her surgeons decided to do a tonsillectomy, adenoidectomy, and partial uvulectomy as a measure to relieve the upper airway obstruction. Postoperatively, and the exact time frame is not clear from the press reports, she bled from the operative site. As a result, she developed intermittent laryngospasm as well as aspirating an unknown quantity of blood into the lungs. Multiple attempts at tracheal intubation were unsuccessful probably because of blood coating all of the oropharyngeal structures making visualization of the larynx impossible. In addition, the girl was no doubt struggling mightily to breathe, with laryngospasm probably also playing a factor. The end result was severe hypoxemia from airway obstruction and cardiac arrest. Ultimately, a tracheal tube was inserted and cardiac function restored. However, she sustained irreversible neurologic brain injury and clinical brain death.

This report reminded one of the authors of another similar event that occurred almost 50 years ago. A 28-year-old man came into the emergency room of a San Francisco hospital complaining of chest pain and difficulty breathing. A chest X-ray was obtained which showed a small wedge-like infarct of the lung. On history, the patient stated that he had injured his right leg playing touch football with his son about a week earlier. On examination it was determined that he had a thrombosis of a leg vein, which was the source of the pulmonary embolism. He was placed on heparin therapy and advised to return every day for evaluation of his coagulation status. Subsequently, he missed his appointments for several days because of a cold. When he returned to the emergency room, he complained of pain in his throat and difficulty swallowing. The emergency room physician did not see anything on examination of his mouth or neck, so sent him to radiology for neck X-rays. He also called the chief resident in anesthesia and asked that he see the patient and offer any advice regarding etiology or treatment.

After completion of the X-rays, the anesthesia resident took a tongue depressor and flashlight and looked in the patient's mouth. At that instant a large volume of blood erupted from the patient's mouth and the patient fell to the floor. Emergency equipment was obtained and the resident attempted bag-mask ventilation with little success. He could not obtain a tight mask fit because of blood on the patient's face. He attempted tracheal intubation by direct laryngoscopy multiple times and then by a blind nasotracheal approach. Each time he inserted a tube into the mouth or nose, blood poured out of the tube. Ultimately he was able to insert an orotracheal tube, but by that time the patient had sustained a substantial period of hypoxemia requiring cardiopulmonary resuscitation. His heart continued to function but he was diagnosed with irreversible brain injury. Mechanical ventilation was terminated a few days later and he died. At autopsy a large, ruptured, upper airway hematoma was diagnosed.

This case was subsequently presented at anesthesia grand rounds at the University of California, San Francisco. The senior faculty was uniformly in agreement that it was futile to spend any appreciable time attempting tracheal intubation. Instead, they advised that the resident should have gone almost immediately to an emergency cricothyrotomy. Over the intervening 50 years the message has not changed.

When bleeding of any magnitude occurs in the naso or oropharynx or upper airway, little or no time should be spent attempting tracheal intubation. Those caring for the patient must go directly to an emergency cricothyrotomy, using a knife or scissors, not a needle. This is the only technique that offers hope for uninjured survival of the patient, and is what should have been done in the Oakland Children's Hospital girl cited above. We know that an emergency cricothyrotomy was not done in her case because it was reported several days after the event that a tracheostomy was considered, but the surgeons stated that such an operation was not indicated in a dead person.

It is imperative that all anesthesia personnel not only know when a cricothyrotomy is the first line of therapy, but also how to perform one quickly. An emergency cricothyrotomy is a very low risk operation even in inexperienced hands, and something that anyone who regards him or herself as an airway expert should be able to do quickly and effectively. Simulation training may provide practitioners the essential skills to perform this procedure when appropriate without concern or fear of causing permanent injury. The Stanford Department of Anesthesiology offers an annual 2-day intensive airway management course that includes hands on instruction using porcine tracheas as the model for a surgical approach to the airway. This training is required for all Stanford anesthesia residents, and should be made available to all anesthesia trainees and anesthesia providers who have not had such training.

Summary

It is essential that every anesthesia provider know both when and how to do an emergency cricothyrotomy. When patients in an operating room or intensive care unit develop severe respiratory insufficiency and hypoxemia that cannot be corrected by bag-mask ventilation or ventilation via an LMA, and immediate tracheal intubation fails, the anesthesia provider must be prepared to perform a 30 s cricothyrotomy. Likewise, acute airway bleeding resulting in respiratory insufficiency can only be treated with an emergency cricothyrotomy. In morbidly obese patients it may be necessary to hyperextend the head and bluntly dissect overlying tissue or blood clot to identify the cricothyroid membrane. Anesthesia providers should regularly palpate the thyroid and cricoid cartilages of anesthetized patients to familiarize themselves with these structures so they can find them quickly in an emergency.

Chapter 7
Bronchospasm vs. Bronchoconstriction: A Different View

Introduction

There is a well-known adage, which says "all that wheezes is not asthma". It is equally true that "all that wheezes during anesthesia is not bronchospasm". It is a widely held view among anesthesia providers that bronchospasm is relatively common during anesthesia. If a large audience of anesthesia providers is asked "How many of you have experienced a case of bronchospasm?" virtually everyone's hands will go up. If they are asked how many have seen multiple cases of bronchospasm, most will raise their hands again. Most anesthesia providers believe that patients with a history of asthma or other bronchospastic disorder have persistent airway hyperreactivity, which may result in intense bronchospasm during anesthesia [1, 2]. We do not share these views. One of the authors has never seen a documented case of bronchospasm in over 50+ years of clinical practice. He has seen many cases where it was thought that bronchospasm was occurring, but on careful examination it proved to be the wrong diagnosis. In our opinion, bronchospasm is a relatively rare cause of wheezing during anesthesia, and because of this fact, it is one of the most **misunderstood**, **misdiagnosed**, and **mistreated** conditions in clinical anesthesia.

When managing a patient under general anesthesia who develops wheezing and requires increased airway pressures to maintain adequate ventilation, the first diagnosis the anesthesia provider should consider is **partial airway obstruction**. Kinking of the tracheal tube or partial occlusion of the tube with secretions or blood may produce wheezing-like sounds during ventilation along with elevation of peak airway pressure. The first step in diagnosis and treatment is to deflate the tracheal tube cuff, suction the tracheal tube, perhaps rotate the tube 45° and establish that it is functioning properly. Once that is done the anesthesia provider should direct attention to passive or active bronchoconstriction.

Both active and passive forces regulate airway size. A decrease in airway size may be caused by either active or passive forces (Table 7.1).

© Springer International Publishing Switzerland 2017
C.P. Larson Jr., R.A. Jaffe, *Practical Anesthetic Management*,
DOI 10.1007/978-3-319-42866-6_7

Table 7.1 Increased airway resistance during anesthesia forces

	Forces	
	Passive	Active
Incidence	Common	Rare
Etiology	Loss of lung volume	Histamine release
		Stimulation airway receptors
Decreased breath sounds	Yes	Yes
Wheezing present	Yes	Yes
Decreased lung compliance	Yes	Yes
Increased peak airway pressure	Yes	Yes
Abdominal wall muscle tone	Increased	Unchanged
Treatment	Increase lung volume	Albuterol aerosol
	Deepen anesthesia	Deepen anesthesia
		Epinephrine if anaphylaxis
Bronchodilators helpful	No	Yes
NMB drugs helpful	Yes	No

There are two active forces which either directly or indirectly cause an increase in smooth muscle tone of the airways to produce constriction. One of the active forces is the autonomic nervous system. The airways are richly innervated by the parasympathetic nervous system, which plays a major role in the constriction of the airways. It is believed that stimulation of irritant receptors in the large airways, for example by the insertion of a tracheal tube, causes a release of acetylcholine from parasympathetic nerves that stimulates M_2 and M_3 muscarinic receptors in airway smooth muscle causing bronchoconstriction [2, 3]. However, this bronchoconstrictive reflex is easily interrupted by anesthetics. For example, the afferent limb is readily blocked by the topical application of local anesthetics in the airway. As well, the efferent limb is blocked by atropine, and the entire reflex is attenuated by general anesthesia or systemically-administered local anesthetics. Hickey et al. showed in dogs that 0.5 MAC halothane blocked vagal bronchoconstriction induced by electrical stimulation of the vagus nerve [4]. Sevoflurane, isoflurane, and halothane have all been shown to be effective bronchodilators at low concentrations.

The second active force regulating airway size is chemical. The most important chemical mediator is histamine, which is contained in mast cells in the airways. Histamine released by anesthetic drugs acts on H_1 receptors in the airway to cause bronchoconstriction of airway smooth muscle. The most dramatic and very rare form of this is anaphylaxis, which within 5 min of administration of the offending anesthetic drug is manifest by wheezing (bronchospasm), decrease in pulmonary compliance, marked decrease in blood pressure, and bradycardia. If not treated promptly with epinephrine, a cardiac arrest may occur. The neuromuscular blocking drugs rocuronium and vecuronium are the most common anesthetic drugs causing anaphylaxis.

Both alpha and beta₂ receptors are present in airway smooth muscle. Stimulation of alpha receptors causes airway constriction, but the reflex is weak and probably not important in the regulation of airway size. Stimulation of beta₂ receptors, for example by circulating epinephrine, activates adenyl cyclase to increase the concentration of cyclic AMP, which in turn causes relaxation of airway smooth muscle [2]. Beta adrenergic blocking drugs (e.g. propranolol) will block this reflex and this may be the mechanism for bronchoconstriction observed in some patients given these drugs. Whether inhalation anesthetics cause bronchodilatation by stimulation of beta$_2$ receptors is not known, but there is evidence that ketamine may cause bronchodilatation by this mechanism. Instead it is generally accepted that inhalation anesthetics act directly on airway smooth muscle to produce bronchodilatation. Maximum dilatation will occur at 0.5 MAC or less.

Normal patients and even most patients who have a history of asthma or other bronchospastic disorders have normal airway resistance when the disease is in remission. At normal lung volumes, airways are at or near maximal dilatation and measurements of airway resistance are in the normal range of 1 cmH$_2$O/L/s. or less. Because of this, the administration of bronchodilator drugs does not increase airway size or decrease airway resistance.

What is not widely recognized or appreciated is that **the single most important determinant of airway size is lung volume**. As lung volume increases during spontaneous ventilation, the increasing negative intrathoracic pressure and expanding alveoli apply radial traction on all of the airways and they enlarge. During mechanical ventilation, positive airway pressure causes airway expansion. With this change, airway resistance decreases and airway conductance (the reciprocal of resistance) increases [5]. Even the large airways such as the trachea and major bronchi enlarge. The reverse occurs as lung volume decreases. The decrease in intrathoracic pressure and loss of radial traction on the airways cause them to narrow. The greater the loss in lung volume, the more constricted the airways become. Briscoe and Dubois demonstrated in 26 patients of varying size and age that there was a close correlation between lung volume and airway resistance and airway conductance (Fig. 7.1) [6].

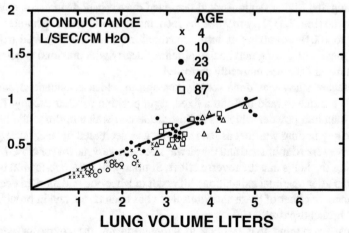

Fig. 7.1 The relationship between age and airway conductance and airway resistance in five subjects each studied at various lung volumes. From Ref. [6]. Reprinted with permission from American Society for Clinical Investigation

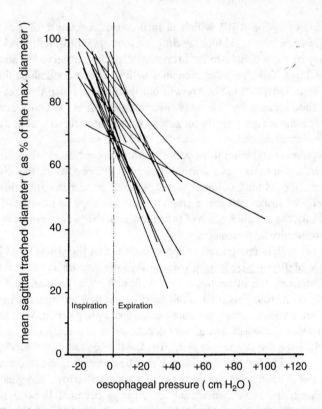

Fig. 7.2 Effect of changes in esophageal pressure induced by maximal inspiration and maximal expiration on intrathoracic tracheal diameter in 19 healthy male patients. From Ref. [7]. Reprinted with permission of the American Thoracic Society. Copyright © 2016 American Thoracic Society

Tammeling and Sluiter demonstrated that even the tracheal diameter is affected by lung volume (Fig. 7.2) [7]. In 19 healthy men, intrathoracic tracheal diameter ranged from 80 to 100 % of maximum during maximal inspiration, and ranged from 20 to 60 % of maximum during maximal expiration. Clearly with maximal exhalation tracheal diameter becomes markedly narrowed.

An elegant study was done some years ago in which anesthetized dogs were placed in a frame to hold them in a fixed, rigid position for fluoroscopy. The dogs inhaled tantalum powder which is radio-opaque and which outlined the bronchial tree. The key finding was that as lung volume was decreased by chest strapping the dogs, airway size diminished and the airways became very narrow or closed entirely. Expanding the lungs had the reverse effect. Similarly, in man, application of a tight chest strap after maximal exhalation will result in wheezing and marked decrease in compliance. In either of these situations there has been no change in bronchomotor tone or "bronchospasm".

Almost everything that is done to patients during the course of general or regional anesthesia results in a loss of lung volume. There are many published studies documenting loss of lung volume with general anesthesia. Preoperative sedation, placement in the supine position, administration of anesthetic drugs, especially neuromuscular blocking agents, and opening the airway to atmospheric pressure during tracheal intubation all result in an elevation of the diaphragm and loss of lung volume. Then a standard tidal volume is instituted. It is important to recognize that tidal volume **is not** lung volume. In this common scenario, whatever tidal volume is instituted is starting at a decreased lung volume. If the decrease in lung volume is substantial, as it may be in patients placed in lithotomy or Trendelenburg position, or patients with an enlarged abdomen from obesity, an intra-abdominal mass, pregnancy or because of restrictive lung disease, the end result is a decrease in lung volume sufficient to cause a severe decrease in airway diameter and its manifestation as wheezing and decreased lung compliance. The clinical interpretation is usually "bronchospasm", but in fact there has been no change in airway muscle tone. A review of published case reports of "bronchospasm" indicated that very few authors considered loss of lung volume as a possible cause, and did not exclude it before calling the condition "bronchospasm" [8–11]. In each report, the cause of the bronchospasm was assigned, but no consideration was given to the possibility that the patient may have lost lung volume.

Several large studies report an incidence of bronchospasm ranging from 0.8 to 20 % in patients with a history of asthma [12–14]. The large variability is thought to be due primarily to different severities of asthma in the study populations. However, there is no indication in any of these studies that the investigators made a careful and systematic analysis of whether the cause of the bronchospasm might be due to loss of lung volume instead of assuming that the cause was bronchospasm because of the history of asthma.

Loss of lung volume can also occur during regional anesthesia. Spinal or epidural anesthesia to a level of T 8 or higher in a patient with a large abdomen may cause marked elevation of the diaphragm and the clinical picture of "bronchospasm". Bronchospasm has been reported during regional anesthesia under circumstances that would suggest that the precipitating cause was loss of lung volume, not "spasm" of the airway smooth muscle [15].

A classic example of "bronchospasm" is the scenario in which general anesthesia is induced in an adult male with a longstanding history of smoking. The induction drugs are propofol or thiopental followed by succinylcholine. Either prior to or after successful tracheal intubation, an inhalation anesthetic is administered. Several minutes later the anesthesia provider notes wheezing and marked difficulty with manual ventilation of the patient's lungs. Attempts are made at deepening anesthesia with sevoflurane, isoflurane, desflurane or propofol and simultaneous administration of aerosolized albuterol to overcome the "bronchospasm". Over time the patient's condition gradually improves, the wheezing stops and peak airway pressure returns to a more normal value with manual or mechanical ventilation. What has actually happened is that the tracheal intubation has stimulated the irritant receptors in the airway, and because of inadequate anesthesia and resolving neuromuscular blockade, the patient reacts by contracting the abdominal muscles, as in a cough or "bucking", thereby markedly decreasing lung volume. Administration of a non-depolarizing neuromuscular blocking drug such as rocuronium or vecuronium will relax the abdominal musculature and improve ventilation. Of course, neither drug has any effect on smooth muscle in the airway, so the original diagnosis of "bronchospasm" was faulty. The problem was loss of lung volume, not spasm of the airway muscles. The inhalation anesthetic would readily overcome any tendency of the airway smooth muscles to contract, as these drugs are potent bronchodilators at low doses. This sequence of events is seen less often as anesthesia providers use longer acting non-depolarizing drugs for tracheal intubation.

The manufacturer voluntarily removed the neuromuscular blocking drug, rapacuronium, from clinical use after several case reports of bronchospasm following tracheal intubation in both children and adults. None of the case reports confirmed that there was no loss of lung volume before diagnosing bronchospasm [16, 17]. Subsequently, Jooste et al. observed that rapacuronium had a higher affinity for the M2 than the M3 muscarinic receptors in Chinese hamster ovary cell culture membranes [3]. They concluded that rapacuronium may potentiate bronchoconstriction by blocking M2 receptors on prejunctional parasympathetic nerves, thereby releasing acetylcholine causing M3 muscarinic receptor-mediated smooth muscle constriction. While this observation may be true, it may have nothing to do with the reports in patients of "bronchospasm", which in reality was decreased airway diameter from loss of lung volume.

The reason that it is important to distinguish between increased airway resistance due to loss of lung volume and that due to airway smooth muscle spasm is because the treatments are different. The treatment for volume-related decreased airway diameter is directed toward increasing lung volume, and the most effective drug will be a neuromuscular blocking agent to relax skeletal muscles, along with augmenting tidal volume and instituting positive end expiratory pressure (PEEP) or continuous positive airway pressure (CPAP). The primary treatment for airway smooth muscle spasm is aerosolized bronchodilators or epinephrine in the rare case of anaphylaxis. In addition, whether the increased airway resistance is due to loss of lung volume or bronchospasm, deepening the level of anesthesia will shorten the duration of the constriction.

Summary

Wheezing and the need for markedly increased airway pressures to maintain effective ventilation occur with some frequency during general anesthesia. When facing this scenario, the first thing to do is to establish that the tracheal tube is functioning properly by deflating the cuff and suctioning its full length to resolve or exclude partial airway obstruction from secretions, blood or kinking of the tube. Once that is done, and the clinical findings persist, consideration should be given to passive increase in airway resistance or active bronchoconstriction.

Increased airway resistance due to loss of lung volume is far more common during general or regional anesthesia than is bronchoconstriction due to spasm of airway smooth muscles, even when the precipitating factor seems to be tracheal intubation. Therefore, the anesthesia provider should direct efforts toward determining if lung volume has decreased substantially due to coughing or bucking and correct it by deepening the level of anesthesia and possibly administering a neuromuscular blocking drug. The anesthesia provider should not waste valuable time administering a bronchodilator, as it will rarely be of benefit. If anaphylaxis is suspected because of the sudden onset of bronchoconstriction and circulatory insufficiency, immediate therapy with epinephrine 0.05–0.1 µg/kg/min should be administered intravenously.

References

1. Pizov R, Brown RH, Weiss YS, Baranov D, Hennes H, Baker S, Hirshman CA. Wheezing during induction of general anesthesia in patients with and without asthma. Anesthesiology. 1995;82:1111–6.
2. Hirshman CA. Airway reactivity in humans: anesthetic implications. Anesthesiology. 1983;58: 170–7.
3. Jooste E, Klafter F, Hirshman CA, Emala CW. A mechanism for rapacuronium-induced bronchospasm: M2 muscarinic receptor antagonism. Anesthesiology. 2003;98:906–11.
4. Hickey RF, Graf PD, Nadel JA, Larson CP. The effects of halothane and cyclopropane on total pulmonary resistance in the dog. Anesthesiology. 1969;31:334–43.
5. Larson CP, Nadel JA. Relationship between airway conductance and airway volume in man. Fed Proc. 1963;22:340.
6. Briscoe WA, Dubois AB. The relationship between airway resistance, airway conductance and lung volume in subjects of different age and body size. J Clin Invest. 1958;37:1279–85.
7. Tammeling GJ, Sluiter HJ. The influence of lung volume, flow rate, and esophageal pressure on the sagittal diameter of the trachea in patients with and without airway obstruction. Am Rev Respir Dis. 1965;92:919–31.
8. Gold MI. Treatment of bronchospasm during anesthesia. Anesth Analg. 1975;54:783–6.
9. Johnson EB, Gold MI. Bronchospasm during pelvic surgery: prostaglandin-kinin pathogenesis? Anesth Analg. 1983;62:104–8.
10. Durant PAC, Joucken K. Bronchospasm and hypotension during cardiopulmonary bypass after preoperative cimetidine and labetalol therapy. Br J Anaesth. 1984;56:917–9.
11. Cooley DM, Glosten B, Roberts JR, Eppes PD, Barnes RB. Bronchospasm after intramuscular 15-methyl prostaglandin F_{2a} and endotracheal intubation in a nonasthmatic patient. Anesth Analg. 1991;73:87–9.
12. Olsson GL. Bronchospasm during anesthesia. A computer-aided incidence study of 136,929 patients. Acta Anaesthesiol Scand. 1987;31:244–52.
13. Kumeta Y, Hattori A, Mimura M, Kishikawa K, Namiki A. A survey of perioperative bronchospasm in 105 patients with reactive airway disease. Masui. 1995;44:396–401.
14. Warner DO, Warner MA, Barnes RD, Offord KP, Schroeder DR, Gray DT, Yunginger JW. Perioperative respiratory complications in patients with asthma. Anesthesiology. 1996;85: 460–7.
15. Mallampati SR. Bronchospasm during spinal anesthesia. Anesth Analg. 1981;60:839–40.
16. Naguib M. How serious is the bronchospasm induced by rapacuronium? Anesthesiology. 2001;94:924–5.
17. Meakin GH, Pronske EH, Lerman J, Orr R, Jaffe D, Savaree AM, Lynn AM. Bronchospasm after rapacuronium in infants and children. Anesthesiology. 2001;94:926–7.

Chapter 8
Management of the Full Stomach

Introduction

Protection of the airway during induction, maintenance and recovery from anesthesia is essential to avoid the consequences of pulmonary aspiration, which can be devastating for both the patient and anesthesia provider. Aspiration of clear liquid secretions from the oropharynx into the airway, so called "silent aspiration" is probably relatively common (although an accurate incidence is not known), and harmless. Of greater concern is the aspiration of regurgitated liquid and/or solid matter from the stomach. Fortunately this type of aspiration is relatively rare, which can lead those providing general anesthesia into complacency, and failure to recognize those circumstances that may promote aspiration.

Incidence of Pulmonary Aspiration

The most comprehensive analysis of this event in adults is contained in a retrospective study published by Warner and colleagues [1]. They defined pulmonary aspiration as "either the presence of bilious secretions or particulate matter in the tracheobronchial tree" or "a postoperative chest X-ray with infiltrates not identified by preoperative chest X-ray or physical examination". Pulmonary aspiration occurred in 67 of 172,335 patients who underwent 215,488 general anesthetics, which gives an incidence of 1:3216 anesthetics.

Based on these Mayo Clinic statistics, the average anesthesia provider administering 600 general anesthetics a year would encounter one pulmonary aspiration about every 5 years.

However, the chances of pulmonary aspiration increase for anesthesia providers who have a larger than usual number of emergency anesthetics (1:895) or patients rated as ASA IV or V (1:1401), but for most providers that would still mean less than

© Springer International Publishing Switzerland 2017   59
C.P. Larson Jr., R.A. Jaffe, *Practical Anesthetic Management*,
DOI 10.1007/978-3-319-42866-6_8

one aspiration per year. This study and others all indicate that pulmonary aspiration is an infrequent occurrence. Of the patients in the Warner study who aspirated, about half (24 of 52) of those undergoing elective surgery and all of the emergency patients (15) had one or more preoperative conditions that are thought to predispose to aspiration, including bowel obstruction, obesity, preoperative opiate administration, depressed consciousness, and ingestion of a meal within 3 h. Aspiration occurred during induction of anesthesia or endotracheal intubation in 57 of the 67 cases, despite the use of cricoid pressure in all cases where aspiration was considered a possibility. Does this mean that cricoid pressure was ineffective in preventing aspiration? This issue will receive greater consideration later in this chapter.

Consequences of Pulmonary Aspiration

In many cases, pulmonary aspiration causes little or no sequellae. In the Warner study 64 % (42 of 66) patients did not develop any symptoms related to the event, and their recovery was uneventful. The remainder (24) developed symptoms and signs of pulmonary aspiration within 2 h of the event. These included cough, wheezing, decrease in arterial oxygen saturation breathing room air, and X-ray evidence of pulmonary aspiration. Of the 24 patients, 18 required special respiratory or intensive care, and 13 required mechanical ventilation. Six patients developed adult respiratory distress syndrome (ARDS), and three died of respiratory failure. While the incidence of death was only 1:71,829 anesthetics, when severe, aspiration can be fatal. The four factors that increase the likelihood of death from aspiration are: age and general health; volume of aspiration; acidity of the aspirate; and contents of the aspirate. Patients who are elderly and have existing pulmonary or cardiovascular diseases are at increased risk of death if pulmonary aspiration occurs. Obviously, the greater the volume of aspirate, which is rarely quantifiable in clinical practice, the greater is the risk of death or severe disability. Likewise, the greater the acidity of the aspirate below pH 2.5, the more severe is the damage to the lungs. Finally, aspiration of solid matter that obstructs major airways, or aspiration of highly infectious material such as fecal matter carries a high mortality in any age group.

Importance of Fasting

Of all the measures designed to prevent aspiration of gastric contents during anesthesia, fasting is the most universal and the most important. Recognizing that the rate of gastric emptying after a meal is highly variable, the ASA Practice Guidelines recommend that anesthesia providers advise adults and children not to ingest a light meal within 6 h, a heavy meal within 8 h, and clear liquids within 2 h of an elective operation. For infants, the fasting recommendations are 2 h for clear liquids, 4 h for breast milk, and 6 h for infant formula and non-human milk [2] (Table 8.1).

Table 8.1 ASA practice guidelines for fasting prior to surgery

Clear liquids	2 h
Breast milk	4 h
Non-human milk	6 h
Light solid foods	6 h
Heavy solid foods	8 h

Use of Prophylactic Medications

The use of prophylactic medications such as antacids (sodium citrate), H_2 receptor antagonists (cimetidine, ranitidine), antiemetics (ondansetron, dolasetron), or drugs to enhance gastric emptying or increase lower esophageal sphincter tone (metoclopromide) to prevent or lessen the severity of pulmonary aspiration is controversial. In the Warner study only half of the patients who aspirated had received any prophylactic medication, and the incidence and severity of the aspiration was no different from those who did not receive the medications. Other studies have shown similar results. The ASA Task Force on Preoperative Fasting concluded from their analysis of existing data that there is insufficient evidence that decreasing gastric acidity or gastric volume, or use of antiemetics decreases either the incidence or sequellae of pulmonary aspiration. While existing evidence challenges the value of prophylactic medication with antacids, H_2 receptor antagonists, and drugs that enhance gastric emptying, it is probably advisable to continue to use one or more of them because of the medicolegal consequences of not doing so.

While prophylactic medications may be helpful, the anesthesia provider should not rely on them to prevent or mitigate the effects of pulmonary aspiration.

Gastroesophageal Reflux Disease (GERD)

This condition has come into prominence in the practice of anesthesiology. Whether the patient has symptoms of GERD is asked of everyone who is about to undergo anesthesia. It is defined as the passive movement of gastric contents into the esophagus, and occasionally into the throat causing irritation of the esophageal and oropharyngeal mucosa. Patients may feel a substernal burning sensation, which in the past was often called "heartburn".

What is known about GERD? Unfortunately, not very much! We do know that GERD is very common. Most, if not all patients experience GERD at one time or another, especially going to bed just after overeating, eating fried, fatty or spicy foods, or after excessive consumption of alcohol. According to the National Institutes of Health, more than 60 million American adults experience GERD at least once a month, and 25 million have daily attacks. However, there are no clear criteria to delineate when GERD changes from being a casual, inconsequential event to becoming a disease. Furthermore, GERD is often referred in the anesthesia literature as being mild, moderate or severe, but there are no data to document what constitutes each category. Is severity based on frequency of attacks, volume of reflux, intensity of symptoms, response to medications, or some combination of these?

Gastroenterologists classify GERD on the basis of findings of mucosal damage at esophagoscopy, or by esophageal findings at roentgenography using double contrast barium swallow examinations. However, most patients reporting GERD have never undergone either of these studies. Finally, while the incidence of pulmonary aspiration in patients with GERD has not been studied in detail, history and clinical experience would certainly indicate that these patients rarely have clinically significant aspiration during anesthesia.

Since there is no scientifically established linkage between GERD and pulmonary aspiration during induction of anesthesia, how should we deal with the patient who has a history of GERD? When interviewing such a patient, two questions are key. First, does the patient have GERD when he/she does not eat? If the answer is no, then it becomes a non-issue for those patients who are NPO prior to surgery. Second, are the symptoms of GERD controlled by diet and/or medications (antacids, H_2 receptor blockers or proton pump inhibitors)? If the answer is yes then one should advise the patient to take their usual medication the day of surgery. Most patients with GERD will fall into one or both of these categories, and other measures to prevent aspiration are unnecessary. To do otherwise would mean that almost all patients are candidates for aspiration prevention.

Current knowledge would support the conclusion that only those patients who have symptomatic GERD when fasting or when taking their medication need to be managed as potential candidates for aspiration during induction of anesthesia and endotracheal intubation.

Is tracheal intubation necessary during general anesthesia in all patients who report a history of GERD? Unfortunately, there are few studies to answer this question. Prudence would suggest that patients who are symptomatic when fasting or when taking their medication should have tracheal intubation if general anesthesia is used. For all other patients, there are no clear guidelines. One study demonstrated that esophageal reflux occurred more frequently during general anesthesia in patients in whom an LMA had been inserted than those managed with a facemask, but none exhibited signs of pulmonary aspiration [3].

Hiatal Hernia

Patients with a known hiatal hernia should **always be managed as candidates for pulmonary aspiration** since the volume and contents of the hernia sac are unknown, the sac is usually below the lower esophageal sphincter, but the diaphragmatic contribution to the prevention of reflux is absent, and its contents may readily empty into the esophagus on induction of anesthesia.

Categories of Full Stomach

Patients who are candidates for pulmonary aspiration can be placed into one of two groups. The difference in the two groups is based on intragastric pressure. In patients with a normal intragastric pressure, the stomach may be partially or completely full, but it is usually at one atmosphere pressure since most patients will burp to decrease the pressure to one atmosphere.

Conditions susceptible to pulmonary aspiration
Group 1: normal intragastric pressure

1. Ingestion of a full meal within 6 h of surgery
2. GERD when not eating and uncontrolled by medication
3. Trauma victims requiring emergency surgery
4. Surgery for sudden onset of pain, with or without narcotic treatment
5. Extremes of age undergoing non-elective surgery
6. Hiatal hernia

In the second group the patient's stomach may be at pressures well above one atmosphere, which means that massive aspiration may occur as soon as general anesthesia is induced. The patients with increased intragastric pressure may have a history of recent vomiting, but that will not necessarily adequately decompress the stomach because the cause of the underlying increased intragastric pressure has not been corrected.

Conditions susceptible to pulmonary aspiration
Group 2: increased intragastric pressure

1. Bowel obstruction
2. GI bleeding
3. Abdominal distension due to pregnancy, ascites, abdominal tumor, etc.

Some texts recommend insertion of a gastric tube to decompress the **stomach in all patients** who have eaten in close proximity to emergency anesthesia. However, this recommendation is not practical, feasible, or even documented as necessary in most patients with normal intragastric pressure. However, it is extremely important to consider inserting an oro or nasogastric tube to decompress the stomach **before inducing general anesthesia** in patients with increased intragastric pressure. The objective of using this tube is to make certain that intragastric pressure is not above one atmosphere. Usually patients with a bowel obstruction or GI bleeding will already have a NG tube in place, but if not, it is highly advisable to insert one orally or nasally before starting the induction. If a patient with suspected increased intragastric pressure refuses to allow insertion of such a tube preoperatively, it would be prudent to document that in the chart and have the patient sign it.

Insertion of an oro or nasogastric tube preoperatively is strongly recommended for any patient suspected of having a bowel obstruction or GI bleed.

It has been a longstanding practice to remove a gastric tube prior to induction of anesthesia because of the concern that it may interfer with mask ventilation and that it may act as a wick and allow gastric contents to track along its course into the oropharynx and promote aspiration. However, recent studies in cadavers indicate that this wicking effect does not occur, and that the tube may actually enhance gastric emptying during induction and intubation. Which practice is safer is not yet established.

Although pulmonary aspiration is as uncommon in infants and children as it is in adults, infants with distended stomachs or bowel obstruction are highly susceptible to pulmonary aspiration [4]. Infants have a tendency to swallow large quantities of air and can generate high intra-abdominal pressures during crying or straining, both of which will greatly increase intragastric pressure, making regurgitation and aspiration likely during induction of anesthesia. Furthermore, it may be more difficult to apply effective cricoid pressure in infants compared to children or adults. Therefore, decompression of the stomach with an oral or nasal tube before induction of anesthesia is recommended in those infants with distended stomachs or suspected bowel obstruction.

Preoxygenation

Preoxygenation prior to induction of general anesthesia may cause absorption atelectasis but is advisable in all patients, and is particularly important in patients who are at risk for aspiration. The two keys to rapid, effective preoxygenation are a tight mask fit and a high gas flow. A tight mask fit prevents the ingress of room air. The high flow of oxygen (about 10 L/min) rapidly replaces the air in the patient's lungs (the functional residual capacity or the volume of gas in the lungs at the end of a normal exhalation, which in adults is about 2–3 L), and more importantly the volume of air in the anesthetic circuit, which may be as large as 7–8 L. If these two steps are followed, it doesn't really matter whether the patient takes normal or deep breaths. With this technique, every inhaled breath will contain pure oxygen. In fact, it is preferable that patients **not take deep breaths** because doing so increases the negative pressure under the mask, and increases the likelihood of air entrainment if the mask fit is not perfect. Preoxygenation is complete when the end-tidal oxygen concentration approaches 85–90 %.

Prevention of Pulmonary Aspiration

With respect to aspiration, two events are of concern during the period from the start of induction of general anesthesia until the airway is secured. These are: **active vomiting** and **passive regurgitation**. Active vomiting is best prevented by ensuring that excellent anesthesia and muscle relaxation have been established before instrumenting the airway. This means that the doses of induction agent (propofol, thiopental, etomidate, or ketamine) and neuromuscular blocking drug (succinylcholine or rocuronium) are adequate to induce anesthesia and paralysis of sufficient depth and duration. Patients cannot actively vomit if they are well anesthetized and paralyzed. Obviously the doses of drugs used must be individualized for each patient, but it is important to remember that giving inadequate doses of these agents increases the risk for aspiration. One can make a strong case for using rocuronium instead of succinylcholine for inducing paralysis for intubation of the larynx. In adequate doses, and with adequate general anesthesia, rocuronium generally provides acceptable conditions for intubation within 1 min after administration. Furthermore, if any difficulty with laryngoscopy is encountered, rocuronium provides relaxation for a sufficient time to resolve the problem. In contrast, the sequence of propofol (or thiopental) and succinylcholine may not give the anesthesia provider the needed time to establish the airway. Because propofol (or thiopental) may be rapidly redistributed away from the brain, and because succinylcholine may be rapidly metabolized, the timing of intubation must be perfect each time this technique is used. If it is not, the anesthesia provider may have unacceptable clinical conditions while trying to intubate the larynx. As well, the patient may recover sufficiently to begin active vomiting before intubation can be accomplished, and pulmonary aspiration during active vomiting is not easily prevented with cricoid pressure.

The only reason for not using rocuronium is because of the concern about a difficult intubation. If that is suspected in advance, then awake fiberoptic intubation is the anesthetic technique of choice. If one encounters an unexpected difficult intubation after induction of anesthesia and paralysis with rocuronium, most of these can be resolved with the use of the Cook (Frova) intubating catheter. In the unusual circumstance where both the standard and Cook intubating techniques fail, one can utilize Plan C (a described technique involving fiberoptic assisted intubation through an LMA) while maintaining cricoid pressure [5]. Occasionally it may be necessary to briefly remove cricoid pressure while inserting a laryngeal mask airway or when inserting a fiberoptic tube through the distal portion of the LMA into the larynx.

Passive regurgitation is best managed by effective cricoid pressure regardless of possible lateral esophageal movement (Fig. 8.1). The anesthesia provider must ensure that the assistant doing the pressure has properly identified the cricoid cartilage before starting induction. Once induction has commenced, the assistant should press downward on the cricoid against the esophagus and stable cervical spine **as hard as he/she can** using only forearm muscles, **and hold the pressure until instructed to stop**. No one has enough strength in the forearm to injure the cricoid or supported cervical spine by the firmest pressure possible. It has been suggested that 30–44 N (7–10 lbs) force is optimal, but its application is unrealistic since very few of those asked to apply cricoid pressure will ever have the opportunity to calibrate the pressure in advance of its utilization. Properly applied cricoid pressure (posterior and slightly upward) should not affect visualization of the laryngeal opening during laryngoscopy.

Since the anesthesiologist is relying on cricoid pressure to prevent passive regurgitation, it must be done correctly.

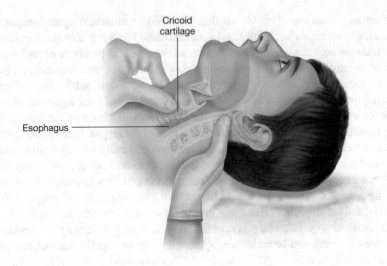

Cricoid
cartilage

Esophagus

Fig. 8.1 Demonstration of how to properly apply cricoid pressure downward as firmly as possible

Reasons for failure of cricoid pressure where failure has occurred have not been clearly documented. In our opinion, failure occurs for one of two reasons: (1) failure to use proper technique; and (2) use of cricoid pressure to prevent aspiration from active vomiting. Cricoid pressure was designed to prevent passive regurgitation; it was never intended nor does it necessarily prevent aspiration from active vomiting. It has been suggested that cricoid pressure decreases lower esophageal tone. If it does, it is irrelevant since one is not relying on sphincter tone to prevent passive regurgitation.

Rapid Sequence Induction

Any plan for anesthetic management of a candidate for aspiration immediately invokes the need for a rapid sequence induction. The term "rapid sequence induction" is the **worst misnomer** in anesthesiology. Unfortunately, it is so imbedded in the lexicon of our specialty that any change in terminology will be difficult to effect. But change is definitely needed! What is wrong with the term? The term "**rapid**" strongly implies that the process from induction of anesthesia to securing the airway with an endotracheal tube must be done quickly, swiftly, or expeditiously. There has never been a study demonstrating any relationship between rapidity of induction (i.e. time from injection of induction drugs to successful intubation of the trachea) and incidence of aspiration. If speed is important, then **both morally and ethically** the most experienced, skilled person at endotracheal intubation who is available should perform the task. However, that is not what is done in clinical practice! Every anesthesia provider in training must learn to manage patients who are candidates for aspiration, so less experienced personnel are routinely allowed and even encouraged to perform the tracheal intubation while the more experienced person supervises. Consequently, the process is not accomplished as rapidly as it could be. Patients and families of patients would be outraged if they knew that "rapid induction and intubation" are considered important, but that the critical task of intubation is being performed by a lesser skilled person while a more skilled person stands by.

A much better term for the whole process is "**safe sequence induction**". This make rapidity no longer an issue, since in reality it is not how rapidly one can accomplish the job but how safely one can do it. Safety during induction and intubation is provided by: (1) insertion of an oro or nasogastric tube for decompression of intragastric pressure where indicated (see above); (2) excellent anesthesia and neuromuscular blockade to prevent active vomiting; and (3) properly applied cricoid pressure to prevent passive regurgitation. Then who performs the intubation or how quickly it is done is no longer an issue.

Another component of a safe sequence induction is ventilation of the lungs while waiting for the induction drugs to take effect. Why is this important? The reasons are twofold. First, gently ventilating the lungs at pressures not exceeding 20 cmH_2O will lessen the risks of hypoxemia and/or hypercapnia if the intubation procedures should be prolonged. Second, knowing that ventilation is possible before starting tracheal intubation is very reassuring that it can be done should intubation prove to be more difficult than anticipated, and more than one attempt is needed. Proper cricoid pressure will prevent any oxygen from entering the stomach during this type of ventilation. If ventilation is difficult during cricoid pressure, directing the cricoid pressure more downward (toward the chest) as well as posterior may help. **There is no documentation that gentle ventilation increases the risk of pulmonary aspiration**.

A recent *in vitro* study suggests that lubrication of the tracheal tube with a water-soluble lubricant lessens the risk of aspiration after tube insertion, perhaps by occluding channels that may exist in the cuff wall. Whether this is of value in patients undergoing surgery who are susceptible to aspiration remains to be demonstrated. Periodic suction of the oropharynx during the anesthetic is also advisable.

Lastly, patients are just as susceptible to pulmonary aspiration during emergence from anesthesia as during induction. Therefore, the tracheal tube must be left in place until airway protective reflexes are intact. This usually means that the patient should be able to respond to commands, and be able to cough vigorously with the tube in place before it is removed.

Summary

Although an uncommon event, pulmonary aspiration continues to occur, and rarely may cause severe disability or death. Therefore, it is important for anesthesiologists to know the conditions that make aspiration more likely, and how to manage them. Preoperative fasting remains a cornerstone for prevention of aspiration. In contrast, the value of prophylactic medications in mitigating the effects of aspiration remains controversial. The relationship of gastroesophageal reflux disease to aspiration is ill defined, and the disease is probably only of importance when it occurs in the absence of eating or drinking or despite taking prophylactic medication. Preoperative insertion of an oro or nasogastric tube is strongly advised when managing a patient with increased intragastric pressure (bowel obstruction, GI bleed, etc.). Effective preoxygenation is always important prior to the induction of anesthesia in patients who are candidates for aspiration. Establishing effective anesthesia and paralysis and utilizing cricoid pressure throughout the interval from induction to tracheal intubation best prevents aspiration. Finally, gentle ventilation of the lungs while waiting for the optimal effects from the induction drugs is recommended. Following these guidelines will result in a "safe sequence induction".

References

1. Warner MA, Warner ME, Weber JG. Clinical significance of pulmonary aspiration during the perioperative period. Anesthesiology. 1993;78:56–62.
2. ASA Task Force on Preoperative Fasting. Practice guidelines for preoperative fasting and the use of pharmacologic agents to reduce the risk of pulmonary aspiration: application to healthy patients undergoing elective procedures: a report by the American Society of Anesthesiologist Task Force on Preoperative Fasting. Anesthesiology. 1999;90:896–905.
3. Ng A, Smith G. Gastroesophageal reflux and aspiration of gastric contents in anesthetic practice. Anesth Analg. 2001;93:494–513.
4. Warner MA, Warner ME, Warner DO, Warner EJ. Perioperative pulmonary aspiration in infants and children. Anesthesiology. 1999;90:66–71.
5. Larson Jr CP. A safe, effective reliable modification of the ASA difficult airway algorithm for adult patients. Curr Rev Clin Anesth. 2002;23:3–12.

Chapter 9
Nitrous Oxide: Yea or Nay

In 1783 Joseph Priestly published his study of a drug that he had prepared, which he called "Dephlogisticated Nitrous Air". His younger friend, Humphrey Davy studied the drug, which he called nitrous oxide, in his laboratory for 2 years and published his findings in 1800. Among his many observations he noted that four or five breaths of nitrous oxide temporarily relieved his headache from indigestion and on another occasion pain from his inflamed gum. In both cases the pain returned after a time but was less intense than originally. Davy's colleagues in chemistry acknowledged his observations but none of them appreciated the fact that it might relieve the pain of surgery. In 1844 a medical student at New York's College of Physicians and Surgeons, Gardner Quincy Colton found that he could earn money for his medical school expenses by attracting patrons into a rented hall and having them inhale nitrous oxide in conjunction with a lecture on chemistry. Those inhaling the gas erupted into loud laughter, which amused the audience and greatly enlivened his lecture. Horace Wells, a dentist in Hartford, Connecticut attended one of these lectures, and subsequently asked Colton to administer nitrous oxide to him while a colleague extracted his painful tooth. While Colton continued to administer nitrous oxide for years afterward for dental extractions both in the United States and England, the discovery of ether and subsequently chloroform anesthesia occupied the attentions of those involved in advancing surgical anesthesia. In 1868 Dr. E. Andrews, a Professor of Surgery at Chicago Medical School published a paper indicating that a mixture of nitrous oxide 75 % with oxygen 25 % might be useful for surgical anesthesia, and subsequently used it on some of his surgical patients. With improved methods for delivery of a nitrous oxide–oxygen mixture over the next 50 years the drug became increasingly popular as an adjuvant for clinical anesthesia. The term "balanced anesthesia" came into the anesthesia lexicon to acknowledge the use of nitrous oxide in combination with a sedative-hypnotic (thiopental), an opiate (morphine, meperidine, etc.) and a neuromuscular blocking drug (succinylcholine, D-tubocurarine). It was widely accepted that nitrous oxide was safe for most patients so long as one avoided a hypoxic gas mixture.

In the last 30 years there has been increasing concern that nitrous oxide may not be as safe as originally thought [1]. This is not a new concern. In 1944 Ralph Waters

© Springer International Publishing Switzerland 2017

C.P. Larson Jr., R.A. Jaffe, *Practical Anesthetic Management*,

DOI 10.1007/978-3-319-42866-6_9

wrote that there was a growing tendency to abandon the use of nitrous oxide because of the technical danger of delivering a hypoxic mixture and the fact that it did not produce any skeletal muscle relaxation [2]. Even in 2015 the question still arises each day in the operating rooms across the United States: Shall we use nitrous oxide on this patient or not…yea or nay? This chapter analyzes the advantages and disadvantages of nitrous oxide so that readers can decide for themselves whether there is still a place for this drug in clinical anesthesia.

Advantages of Nitrous Oxide

> **Advantages of Nitrous Oxide**
> Moderate analgesia
> Rapid onset, rapid recovery
> Circulatory support
> Inexpensive
> Safe in patients with known malignant hyperthermia

Analgesia

The most important advantage of nitrous oxide is its ability to produce analgesia in a dose dependent manner, the greater the dose, the greater the analgesic effect. Unfortunately, the upper limit of dosage is 60–70 % concentration to avoid hypoxemia, and at that dose range nitrous oxide does not provide adequate analgesia for surgery. For surgical anesthesia nitrous oxide must be used in combination with other anesthetics such as propofol, opiates (fentanyl, meperidine, dihydromorphone) or inhalation anesthetics (sevoflurane, desflurane or isoflurane). The minimum anesthetic concentration (MAC) for nitrous oxide is 105 %, so at 60 % concentration it decreases the need for other analgesics by about 50 %. However, since the analgesic requirement of patients is so variable, this is only a rough approximation of its analgesic interaction with other drugs.

Insolubility

The second most important advantage of nitrous oxide is its insolubility. Its blood-gas partition coefficient is 0.47, which means that for every molecule of nitrous oxide in the blood phase there are two molecules in the gas phase. This insolubility and the fact that nitrous oxide is both odorless and tasteless render it an excellent drug for inducing general anesthesia by inhalation. Administering nitrous oxide 6–8 L/min flow with oxygen 3–4 L/min flow will induce a quick loss of awareness and allow for the introduction of sevoflurane in a rapidly increasing concentration with minimal or no recall of the odor of sevoflurane, even though it is a pleasant one. A high total gas flow at the start of an inhalation induction anesthetic is essential to quickly replace the air in the 8–10 L anesthetic circuit and patient functional residual capacity as well as to match the large volume of nitrous oxide uptake in the first 5–10 min. Manually augmenting ventilation during this induction phase will greatly increase the speed of induction, since uptake of insoluble anesthetics is enhanced more by ventilation than by circulation. Inhalation induction with nitrous oxide/sevoflurane is by far the safest type of induction of anesthesia since if any untoward events should occur (hypotension, arrhythmia, etc.), the gases can be quickly replaced with pure oxygen. Since there is very little venous or tissue content of nitrous oxide or sevoflurane during induction, the patient will awaken from anesthesia very quickly. Inhalation inductions with nitrous oxide/sevoflurane will become an increasing part of clinical practice in the future as the ability to easily find intravenous access preoperatively becomes more difficult owing to old age, obesity, chemotherapy, etc. General anesthesia generally makes obtaining peripheral intravenous access easier. The insolubility of nitrous oxide also makes it easier to change anesthetic concentrations quickly when compared to other inhaled anesthetics. If one wishes to increase the anesthetic concentration of nitrous oxide from 50 to 60 % or decrease the concentration from 60 % to zero, it can be done very quickly by either using a high gas flow of nitrous oxide 60 % or a high gas flow of oxygen 100 %, and in both cases also augmenting ventilation.

The combination of high total gas flows and rapid transition from spontaneous to manually controlled ventilation will greatly speed up an inhalation induction with nitrous oxide/sevoflurane.

Once anesthesia is induced and the inspired and expired concentrations of nitrous oxide are in equilibrium, nitrous oxide flow can be decreased to 1 L/min or less with a corresponding oxygen flow of 0.8–1 L/min or less to maintain oxygen saturation at 97 % or greater. Since there is no loss of nitrous oxide to metabolism, and only a very small loss over time via the skin, it is acceptable to use even lower flows of nitrous oxide and oxygen if one wishes.

Circulatory Support

Nitrous oxide is a mild myocardial depressant, but stimulates the sympathetic nervous system with consequent maintenance of both cardiac output and blood pressure. In most circumstances this is an advantage, but it can be a disadvantage if one is trying to decrease mean pressure to decrease blood loss at the surgical site. One of the interesting and totally unstudied side effects of nitrous oxide is that when it is combined with meperidine, a bradycardia ensues, usually with heart rates in the range of 50–60 b/min. This interaction is surprising because meperidine is a derivative of atropine, so one would expect a tachycardia instead of a bradycardia. The only time that bradycardia does not occur is when the patient is hypovolemic or if the depth of anesthesia is inadequate for the surgical stimulus. Nitrous oxide is the only inhaled anesthetic that has been shown not to provide cardioprotection as a result of administering it prior to an episode of ischemia (anesthetic preconditioning).

Cost

No consideration of the value of a drug is complete without analysis of its cost relative to alternative drugs. Most anesthetic drugs are purchased under contract with a vendor, and the exact price will vary depending upon such things as the number and volume of drugs purchased from that vendor, shipping costs, etc. As one benchmark, at one institution the cost of sevoflurane 2% delivered in a total gas flow of 2 L/min for 1 h is $ 5.14. This is based on a 250 mL bottle price of $ 93.11. The cost for desflurane 6% delivered at the same flow rate for 1 h is $ 20.47 based on a 240 mL bottle price of $ 142.11. One problem with this comparison is that if an institution does not use much desflurane then the purchase price is higher. The cost of nitrous oxide delivered at a flow rate of 2 L/min for 1 h is $ 0.87. What this illustrates is: (a) the lower the total gas flow rate, the lower the cost of the drug; and (b) nitrous oxide is much less expensive than the commonly used volatile agents. Cost should never be the primary driving force in the selection of anesthetic drugs, but anesthesia providers must be cognizant of the cost savings that can accrue over time by using nitrous oxide in combination with volatile agents rather than using the volatile agents alone.

Disadvantages of Nitrous Oxide

There are several circumstances or transition states where the use of nitrous oxide is inappropriate or highly questionable.

Questionable Use of Nitrous Oxide
During transition states

   Moving patients supine to prone, supine to sitting
   Rotating bed 45, 90 or 180°
   Changing from controlled to spontaneous ventilation

Rib fractures
Pulmonary hypertension
Application of tympanic membrane grafts
Gas injection into the eye during ocular surgery
Harvesting abdominal tissue for tram flaps
Intra-abdominal surgery
Presence of subcutaneous emphysema
History of intractable nausea/vomiting from anesthesia

Transition States

One very common transition state occurs when anesthetized patients are moved from the supine to the sitting or prone positions, or the patient's bed is turned 45, 90 or 180°. In such circumstances one does not know how long the repositioning will take or whether untoward events such as the tracheal tube being moved or dislodged will occur until the move is completed. If controlled ventilation with nitrous oxide 60% is being administered prior to the move, ventilation must resume within 1–2 min to avoid hypoxemia. If instead, oxygen 100% is administered prior to the move, one has 8–10 min to resolve any problems that might occur during the move before hypoxemia occurs. This time difference is substantial and important if one needs to correct a problem with the patient or equipment occurring as a result of the move.

Another transition state occurs near the conclusion of virtually every general anesthetic. If nitrous oxide and sevoflurane or isoflurane have been used for anesthesia, it is common practice to lighten the level of anesthesia by decreasing or turning off the inspired concentration of sevoflurane or isoflurane, and perhaps decreasing the volume of ventilation to increase the concentration of carbon dioxide in the blood, while keeping the concentration of nitrous oxide at 50–60%. The rationale behind this practice relates to the fact that nitrous oxide is less soluble than the two volatile agents, so that when the surgery ends, the patient will emerge from anesthesia faster than if the nitrous oxide is discontinued and the anesthetic maintained until the conclusion of surgery with either of the volatile agents. However, this rationale is flawed and the practice highly questionable especially as applied to sevoflurane. With respect to the rapidity of emergence issue, the blood solubility of sevoflurane is so close to that of nitrous oxide (0.65, 0.47) that the differences in wakeup time are trivial (within 1–2 min of each other). So there is really no significant benefit of nitrous oxide acting as a faster emergence drug.

There are a number of important reasons for not using this practice. First, with the nitrous oxide concentration at 50–60% and controlled ventilation decreased to increase the blood carbon dioxide level, the oxygen saturation will decrease, sometimes to unacceptable levels. Second, as the sevoflurane or isoflurane concentrations, and hence MACs decrease, the patient may cough or buck on the tracheal tube. That will cause an immediate loss of lung volume, and since pulmonary ventilation is decreased more than pulmonary circulation, a right to left shunt will be created in the lungs causing oxygen desaturation. The next inhaled breath will contain nitrous oxide, which will not correct the desaturation regardless of whether the subsequent ventilation is spontaneous, assisted or controlled. To stop the coughing or bucking, the anesthesia provider will have to either remove the tracheal tube or administer an intravenous drug such as propofol or lidocaine. Removing the tracheal tube under these circumstances is unwise. With 50–60% nitrous oxide still in the lungs, allowing the patient to breathe room air is the scenario where diffusion hypoxia occurs. Administering intravenous drugs introduces other problems including failure to stop the coughing/bucking, cessation of spontaneous ventilation, or causing an unacceptable decrease in blood pressure. There is no value to increasing the concentration of sevoflurane or isoflurane at this point to stop the coughing/bucking because the venous and tissue concentrations of the drug have decreased, and it will take a while to re-establish surgical anesthesia. In sum, this practice is misguided, illogical and offers no benefit and substantial risks to patients.

Nitrous oxide offers no advantages and introduces substantial risks when maintained at anesthetic concentrations during emergence from anesthesia.

Instead what should be done during the latter stages of the anesthetic is to turn off the nitrous oxide, increase total oxygen flow to 8–10 L/min and double the inspired concentration of sevoflurane or isoflurane so as to stay at the same MAC value that existed when the nitrous oxide was being administered. Controlled ventilation should be continued until the expired oxygen concentration reaches about 80 %, at which time the oxygen flow should be decreased to 300–400 mL and the ventilator turned off. Carbon dioxide will accumulate in the patient's body, and eventually the patient will start to breathe. Regardless of the time it takes to restore spontaneous ventilation, the patient will not become desaturated because of the continuous mass oxygen flow from the source (flowmeter or reservoir bag) to the alveoli. Only three events would cause desaturation while awaiting spontaneous ventilation, namely circuit disconnect allowing air (nitrogen) into the system; patient biting on the tracheal tube preventing mass movement of oxygen from the source to the lungs; and massive atelectasis with substantial right to left shunting of blood in the lungs. The latter event is uncommon even in morbidly obese patients.

> **Definite Contraindications to Nitrous Oxide Use**
> Hypoxemia breathing room air
> Pneumothorax; pneumocephalus
> Known vitamin B^{12} deficiency
> Abdominal laparoscopic procedures
> Laser airway surgery

Presence of Air Cavities

Because of its dislike for tissue, nitrous oxide will readily diffuse from blood into air cavities that have a blood supply. For example, nitrous oxide will diffuse into the maxillary sinuses and middle ear cavities but this is rarely a problem since these are easily vented. However, when a graft is to be placed on the tympanic membrane, surgeons will ask that nitrous oxide not be used. Nitrous oxide is almost always avoided in abdominal surgery, particularly laparoscopic procedures because of the distension of the bowel that occurs when it is used. For the same reason, surgeons' performing tram flaps will ask that nitrous oxide not be used until the abdominal flap is mobilized and the abdominal wall is closed. Nitrous oxide is contraindicated in any patient with a pathological air cavity such as a pneumothorax or pneumocephalus as that cavity can double or triple in size depending upon the concentration of nitrous oxide being used. It is probably unwise to use nitrous oxide in any patient with rib fractures even if a chest roentgenogram does not show a pneumothorax. Nitrous oxide should probably not be used in patients with evidence of subcutaneous emphysema since those air pockets will enlarge. Nitrous oxide should not be used if a gas pocket is to be placed in the eye. Nitrous oxide will increase the pressure in a tracheal tube cuff inflated with air. This increased pressure may cause irritation or ischemia of tracheal mucosa and postoperative sore throat.

Pulmonary Hypertension

Nitrous oxide should be avoided in patients with pulmonary hypertension or elevated pulmonary vascular resistance because nitrous oxide can produce small but physiologically significant increases in pulmonary artery pressure, pulmonary artery occlusion pressure, and pulmonary vascular resistance.

Prolonged Exposure

Rodents exposed to anesthetic concentrations of nitrous oxide for days or weeks may develop a vitamin B^{12} deficiency as a result of inactivation of methionine synthetase. Inactivation of this enzyme interferes with DNA synthesis and may produce clinical findings characteristic of vitamin B^{12} deficiency. Prolonged exposure of operating room personnel to subanesthetic concentrations of nitrous oxide is no longer an issue since modern operating rooms have efficient air circulation systems, and the anesthetic gases are scavenged to outside of the hospital. There have been a few case reports of patients exposed to anesthetic concentrations of nitrous oxide (50–60 %) for an hour or two developing a clinical picture of a vitamin B^{12} deficiency days or weeks later [3]. The patients complained of weakness, numbness and/or paresthesias in their legs, difficulty walking, blurred vision and mental confusion. Therapy with vitamin B^{12} seemed to improve the patients' conditions so it was assumed that the nitrous oxide was the causative agent. However, in most of these rare case reports there are virtually no descriptions of what transpired from the time of exposure to development of symptoms. What were the patients' background conditions; had they had similar symptoms before being exposed to nitrous oxide; what other drugs were they taking; etc.? In most cases it has the appearance of guilt by association rather than by solid scientific evidence. Many millions (or even billions) of patients have been exposed to nitrous oxide without any adverse sequelae, so concern over vitamin B^{12} deficiency is not a legitimate reason to restrict or abandon the use of the drug. Nitrous oxide should be avoided in the rare patient with known or suspected vitamin B^{12} deficiency.

Laser Surgery

Nitrous oxide supports combustion so it should not be administered when patients are undergoing laser surgery of the airways or lungs.

Special Issues

Nausea/Vomiting

It is well established that patients receiving nitrous oxide have a higher incidence of postoperative nausea and vomiting than those who do not. However, since most of these patients will be receiving other anesthetics such as opiates and volatile anesthetics that are also associated with nausea and vomiting, it seems ironic to single out nitrous oxide as the drug to be avoided. If postoperative nausea and vomiting is the primary issue in selecting anesthetic agents, two options are available. One, either avoid nitrous oxide altogether, or two, administer antiemetics: odansetron or dolasetron as the serotonin receptor antagonist; droperidol or metaclopromide as the dopamanergic receptor antagonist; and dexamethasone as an excellent nonspecific antiemetic, all given near the conclusion of surgery. Additional doses of these drugs are advisable for up to 24 h postoperatively, especially if opiates are to be administered for pain.

Diffusion Hypoxia

If patients are allowed to breathe room air immediately after breathing nitrous oxide 50–70 %, the patients may develop what has been termed "diffusion hypoxia". This is the only circumstance in clinical anesthesia where this occurs. With each breath of room air, patients inhale nitrogen 79 %, and because nitrogen is so insoluble in tissues most of it remains in the lungs. With each exhalation, patients are excreting nitrous oxide, but the volume of nitrous oxide in the body that is available for entry into the lungs is substantial. As a result, the combination of an increasing concentration of nitrogen in the lungs and the presence of a high concentration of nitrous oxide results in a sudden decrease in lung oxygen, which in turn causes transient hypoxemia. Of equal concern is the fact that with diffusion hypoxia, patients will also develop "diffusion hypocapnia". Just as the oxygen in the lungs is diluted, so is the carbon dioxide. The diffusion hypocapnia may, in turn cause hypoventilation, which will worsen both the hypoxemia and hypocapnia. These issues are of particular concern in patients with pre-existing lung disease. Diffusion hypoxia can be avoided by the administration of oxygen for several minutes at a high flow to avoid rebreathing of nitrous oxide prior to allowing patients to breathe room air. This maneuver will not prevent diffusion hypocapnia, but transient hypoventilation is of minimal concern when the lungs contain a high concentration of oxygen.

Malignant Hyperthermia

Nitrous oxide is an acceptable agent for use in patients with a history of malignant hyperthermia. The only concern regarding the use of nitrous oxide in these patients is its ability to stimulate the sympathetic nervous system, which in turn, may cause cutaneous vasoconstriction and thereby limit cutaneous heat loss.

ENIGMA Trials

A large group of multinational investigators have published two randomized control trials comparing outcomes in patients given either 70 % N_2O or 20 % N_2 in oxygen (ENIGMA-I), or 70 % N_2O or 70 % N_2 in oxygen (ENIGMA-II) during 2–4 h surgeries. In ENIGMA-I with 2050 patients equally divided between the two groups, the incidence of severe nausea/vomiting, wound infection, fever, pulmonary complications, and myocardial infarction postoperatively were greater in the nitrous oxide group. However, there was no difference in length of stay in the hospital between the two groups [4]. In ENIGMA-II with another 7000 patients using a similar research protocol, the investigators found that there was no difference in the incidence of myocardial, stroke or death between the two groups [5]. It is not known whether the different outcomes in the two trials were due to the beneficial effects of high concentrations of oxygen. There are compelling reasons for administering high concentrations of oxygen (80 %) during surgery. Patients administered high-inspired oxygen concentrations have a lower incidence of surgical site infections and postoperative nausea and vomiting, with some studies suggesting no significant increase in the incidence of postoperative atelectasis when compared to patients given air or nitrous oxide. However, after very comprehensive review of the published literature, the Cochrane report concluded that during clinical anesthesia "As the risk of adverse events, including mortality, may be increased by a fraction of inspired oxygen of 60 % or higher, and as robust evidence is lacking for a beneficial effect of a fraction of inspired oxygen of 60 % or higher on surgical site infection, our overall results suggest that evidence is insufficient to support the routine use of a high fraction of inspired oxygen during anesthesia and surgery" [6].

The final answer as to if and when to use high concentrations of oxygen in the operative and postoperative phase in patients has not been answered. For sure, high oxygen is desirable during induction and establishment of the airway, but after that each anesthesiologist must make an individual decision whether to continue high oxygen concentrations based on the patient's condition, the operative procedure, the patient responses to the anesthetic, blood loss, and other factors.

GALA Trial

In this study 1615 patients undergoing carotid surgery were nonrandomized into one of two groups: 671 received nitrous oxide (GA) and 944 a regional block (LA) [7]. The GA group had a significantly higher incidence of coronary artery disease, peripheral vascular disease, and atrial fibrillation. Despite this, the use of nitrous oxide did not increase the comparative risk of myocardial infarction, stroke or death within 30 days following surgery.

Greenhouse Gas

It is well known that nitrous oxide is a greenhouse gas that is the major ozone-depleting gas in the twenty-first century. As Baum et al. point out [8], the exhaust of nitrous oxide from scavenging systems into the atmosphere is trivial (<0.05 %) when compared to the exhaust from agricultural activities and other sources. It is something to be aware of, but it is not a dominant reason to avoid using nitrous oxide in anesthesia.

Summary

With the evidence from the Cochrane review [6] that the use of high concentrations of oxygen in the operative and postoperative period is probably more detrimental than beneficial, the use of nitrous oxide or air during routine anesthesia care would seem appropriate. The evidence is also not compelling enough to conclude that it is time to abandon the use of nitrous oxide in clinical anesthesia. There are certainly circumstances where its use is highly questionable or clearly inappropriate (see above). There are also situations where its use is extremely valuable, such as during inhalation inductions in adults and children, in patients with known malignant hyperthermia syndrome, or in circumstances where brief, quick analgesia is needed. In the end, each anesthesia provider must decide whether or not to use nitrous oxide in most patients on the basis of personal beliefs or choice rather than on sound scientific evidence.

References

1. Eger EI, editor. Nitrous oxide/N_2O. New York: Elsevier Science; 1985. p. 1–369.
2. Waters RW. Nitrous oxide centennial. Anesthesiology. 1944;5:551–65.
3. Flippo TS, Holder Jr WD. Neurologic degeneration associated with nitrous oxide anesthesia in patients with vitamin B_{12} deficiency. Arch Surg. 1993;128:1391–5.

4. Miles PS, Leslie K, Chan MTV, Forbes A, Paech MJ, Peyton P, Silbert BS, Pascoe E, and ENIGMA Trial Group. Avoidance of nitrous oxide for patients undergoing major surgery. Anesthesiology 2007;107:221–31.
5. Leslie K, Myles PS, Chan MTV, Forbes A, Paech MJ, Payton P, Silbert BS, Williamson E. Nitrous oxide and long-term morbidity and mortality in the ENIGMA trial. Anesth Analg. 2011;112:387–93.
6. Meyhoff WJ, Jorgensen LN, Gluud C, Lindschon J, Rasmussen LS. The effects of high perioperative inspiratory oxygen fraction for adult surgical patients (review). Reprint of a Cochrane review. Cochrane Libr. 2015;6:1–116.
7. Sanders RD, Graham E, Lewis SC, Gough MJ, Warlow C. Nitrous oxide exposure does not seem to be associated with increased mortality, stroke and myocardial infarction: a non-randomized subgroup analysis of the general anaesthesia compared with local anaesthesia for carotid surgery (GALA) trial. Br J Anaesth. 2012;109:361–7.
8. Baum VC, Willschke H, Marciniak B. Is nitrous oxide necessary in the future? Pediatr Anesth. 2012;22:981–7.

Chapter 10
Meperidine: A Forgotten Jewel

At one time meperidine was the most commonly used opioid for surgical anesthesia or as a supplement to regional anesthesia. Its decline as an operating room analgesic after many years of successful use was the result of at least two events. One was the development of ultra short acting opiates. Fentanyl, synthesized in the late 1960s by Paul Janssen, and later its derivatives sufentanil, alfentanil, and remifentanil, gradually replaced meperidine in the operating rooms of United States hospitals. The general thinking was that shorter acting opiates would be easier and safer to administer and manage than longer acting ones. The other event was that meperidine became an unpopular analgesic drug among clinicians in general medicine and surgery because of its side effects, namely nausea and vomiting, adverse interaction with MAO inhibitor drugs, and normeperidine toxicity causing seizures. The increasing distain for meperidine within medical circles had a strong influence on the anesthesia community. However, the reasons that clinicians were abandoning meperidine were for the most part either specious or irrelevant to its use in clinical anesthesia. For example, there is no evidence that meperidine is more emetogenic than the newer opiates. Further, the MAO inhibitors have been almost completely replaced by more effective drugs that do not have any unique interaction with meperidine. Finally, there has never been a case report or study documenting seizures from the use of meperidine in the operating room. Nevertheless, today meperidine is used almost exclusively as a single dose only treatment for postoperative shivering or as an analgesic for short, outpatient diagnostic procedures. As a result, whole generations of anesthesia providers have not had training in the use of or experience with meperidine. This is very unfortunate because meperidine has properties that make it an excellent operating room analgesic.

© Springer International Publishing Switzerland 2017
C.P. Larson Jr., R.A. Jaffe, *Practical Anesthetic Management*,
DOI 10.1007/978-3-319-42866-6_10

History

Meperidine was the first opioid to be synthesized in the laboratory and in 1939 that was a unique way to create a new drug. In an effort to develop a better vagolytic drug than atropine, two German scientists, Von O. Eisleb and O. Schaumann reconfigured the atropine molecule, and developed several new agents, the most promising of which was one they named "dolantin" [1, 2]. They administered dolantin to both mice and cats and observed that it was a less potent vagolytic than atropine, but much to their surprise it had spasmolytic and analgesic effects. In comparative studies with morphine, they found it to be an effective but less potent analgesic. In comparative studies with codeine, they found that it was as effective as codeine in suppressing tracheal cough reflexes.

In 1943 Rovenstine and Batterman reported on the successful use of meperidine as a preanesthetic medication in 338 patients who were to undergo general anesthesia [3]. Shortly thereafter, Batterman and Himmelsbach reported in patients that meperidine 100 mg produced an analgesic effect equivalent to morphine 10 mg [4]. Following these reports, the drug was gradually introduced into operating room anesthesia as a substitute for morphine as part of a "balanced" anesthetic technique.

Pharmacology

Meperidine (1-methyl 4-phenyl-piperidine 4-carboxylic acid ethyl ester hydrochloride) is a member of the phenylpiperidine series, which includes fentanyl, sufentanil, alfentanil and remifentanil. Meperidine chemical structure is very similar to that of atropine and quite different from morphine (Fig. 10.1). As a result, it is not surprising that it has some of the same pharmacological effects as atropine. For example, it has a mild antimuscarinic effect manifested as a slight increase in heart rate. When initially studied, it was thought that meperidine had a mild spasmolytic effect on smooth muscle which would provide some suppression of coughing when the tracheal mucosa is irritated, as well as relaxing gastric and bowel smooth muscle thereby delaying gastric emptying and decreasing bowel motility. Because of its relaxant effect on airway smooth muscle, early investigators thought that it might be a useful drug for treating patients with bronchial asthma, but that did not prove to be the case. More recent studies have also shown that the spasmolytic effects on smooth muscle are minimal, and probably not of therapeutic benefit. However, it has two effects that are not characteristic of atropine, namely sedation and analgesia. Meperidine will produce mild sedation and euphoria, both of which make it a useful drug as a premedicant for patients undergoing regional anesthesia or diagnostic procedures under monitored anesthesia care. More importantly, meperidine is an effective analgesic because of its action on the μ receptors, and to a lesser extent on the δ and k receptors in the central nervous system. Because of its analgesic property, it was the most commonly used opiate in clinical anesthesia for more than 20 years until fentanyl was developed.

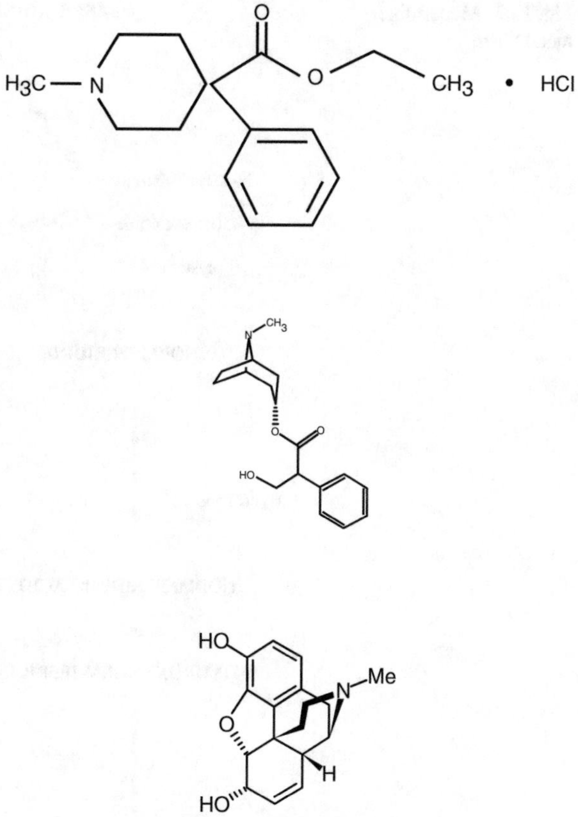

Fig. 10.1 Chemical structures of meperidine (*top*), atropine (*center*) and morphine (*bottom*)

Meperidine is somewhat less lipid soluble than fentanyl, so its onset of action following intravenous administration is about 5 min compared to 1–3 min for fentanyl. Meperidine duration of action from a single dose is about 2–3 h. Meperidine has a large volume of distribution and 65–75 % is protein bound. Meperidine undergoes relatively rapid metabolism in the liver via two routes, the predominant pathway being hydrolysis to form meperidinic acid, and the lesser pathway being N-demethylation to form the active metabolite normeperidine (Fig. 10.2). Normeperidine then undergoes hydrolysis in the liver to form normeperidinic acid. Both acid forms are inactive and are excreted by the kidneys. Animal studies have demonstrated that normeperidine has an analgesic potency about half of its parent compound. However, accumulation of normeperidine (elimination half-life 15–30 h) may cause central nervous system irritability as manifest by myoclonic jerks and seizures. Evidence that the same may occur in humans is entirely circumstantial, based on case reports of patients developing nervousness, dysphoria, tremors, myoclonus and occasionally seizures after having received meperidine for days or weeks as a treatment for chronic pain. However, there is no clear relationship between normeperidine toxicity and CNS irritability and seizures in patients.

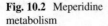

Fig. 10.2 Meperidine
metabolism

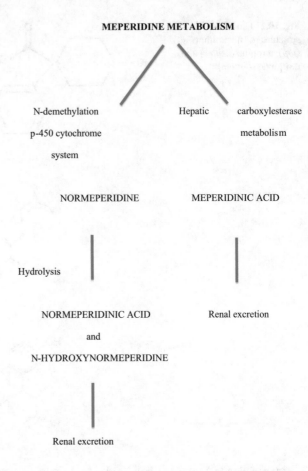

Manifestations of toxicity are most likely to occur in patients receiving meperidine in high doses (>1000 mg/24 h), for prolonged periods (days to weeks), or those patients in renal failure, which may prolong the normal renal excretion of normeperidine. Normeperidine toxicity has never been an issue with the use of meperidine in operating room anesthesia because the doses of meperidine used as part of a balanced anesthesia technique are too low (less than 300–400 mg) and too short a duration of administration (much less than 24 h) to produce normeperidine neurotoxicity even in patients in renal failure. There has never been a documented case of a seizure due to meperidine when administered as an adjuvant in clinical anesthesia.

In some patients, meperidine may cause a histamine reaction, most commonly manifested as cutaneous redness and blotching around the vein at the site of an intravenous injection. This may cause some itching specifically at the injection site. Nasal itching is also common, but it is not known whether the mechanism is histamine release or a central mechanism. These are trivial events, do not require treatment, and subside in a few minutes. It has been suggested that meperidine is associated with significant histamine release, and should be used cautiously in patients with a history of asthma [5, 6]. However, the authors did not provide any definition of "significant", or provide any case reports documenting an asthmatic event due to meperidine. In our extensive use of meperidine, the histamine reactions have always been local, never systemic. This is another example of how an undocumented postulate becomes "fact" and alters medical care.

Usually there are no cardiovascular changes associated with intravenous meperidine injections unless a very large dose (100 mg) is given as a single bolus. The hypotension from such large doses is probably due to myocardial depression with or without some vascular dilatation from histamine release.

Respiratory depression is a feature of all opiates, and meperidine is no exception. The respiratory depression is dose related and is no worse or better than other opiates. With increasing doses, meperidine causes a progressive decrease in respiratory rate and increase in tidal volume, with the net effect being a decrease in minute and alveolar ventilation and increasing arterial and end-tidal carbon dioxide. If used in combination with a volatile anesthetic such as sevoflurane or isoflurane, tidal volume decreases instead of increasing, so alveolar ventilation is decreased even more. However, unless given in very large bolus doses, meperidine will not cause cessation of breathing or apnea. In contrast to meperidine, fentanyl and its derivatives may cause apnea even in small doses (50–100 µg) and even in healthy patients. This difference has important implications in the selection of an opiate as a premedicant or for treatment of acute postoperative pain in the postanesthesia care unit. For example, orthopedic patients who come to hospital for surgery are often in pain and accustomed to taking one or more of a variety of analgesics. Usually they are instructed not to take any analgesics the day of surgery so they arrive in the preoperative suite complaining of pain. Nurses in the unit then call the anesthesia provider requesting an order for an analgesic. Meperidine is an ideal drug in this circumstance. A dose of 20–25 mg can be administered safely intravenously and it will alleviate the pain within 10 min. If after 15 min the patient is still complaining (probably because of opiate tolerance), a second, similar dose can be administered safely. Doses administered in this manner will not make the patient apneic. The same drug scenario can be used for patients experiencing acute pain in the postanesthesia care unit. Many anesthesia providers would use fentanyl in these circumstances, but we would strongly recommend against it. Fentanyl may cause sudden apnea, and if not detected immediately may cause hypoxemia, hypotension and even cardiac arrest. We would urge that anesthesia providers not order fentanyl or its derivatives in any setting other than those where the provider can watch the patient for at least 15–20 min after its administration. We know of a case where fentanyl was administered to a patient in pain, put into a CT scanner, and when removed from the scanner the patient was dead, or where emergency room patients were given fentanyl to reduce a fracture or suture a wound, and when they returned to do the procedure, the patients were dead. Likewise, we have seen multiple cases of acute apnea following administration of fentanyl in a recovery room, but fortunately none of them resulted in permanent injury.

Acute tolerance will occur after the administration of multiple doses of meperidine, so its effectiveness in managing pain wanes over 24–48 h. With repeated administration it may also cause psychic and physical dependence in some patients, and its addiction potential is probably equivalent to that of morphine or fentanyl and its derivatives.

Meperidine is a potent alpha 2 agonist [7] and like clonidine is very effective in abolishing shivering, and more importantly, decreasing oxygen consumption from the shivering in patients who are recovering from general or regional anesthesia. The finding that other opioid drugs are not effective in treating shivering, and that butorphanol (a kappa receptor agonist-antagonist) is effective suggests that its mechanism of action may be due in part to its effect on the k-opioid receptors in the CNS. However, the evidence that this is the mechanism is very circumstantial. While other drugs may resolve postoperative shivering, meperidine is the drug of choice because of its availability, ease of administration, and effectiveness.

Meperidine should not be administered to patients who are taking monoamine oxidase inhibitor drugs (MAOI's) such as isocarboxazid (Marplan), phenelzine sulfate (Nardil), or tranylcypromine sulfate (Parnate). An interaction between these drugs and meperidine may cause an excess release of serotonin (5 HT) and/or a delay in its reuptake in the central nervous system causing a "serotonin syndrome", which might be manifested as fever, shivering, diaphoresis or myoclonus in the anesthetized patient. Serotonin syndrome can also occur with any of the other phenvipiperidine derivatives including fentanyl and sufentanil when administered to patients on non-MAOI antidepressants. This is very rarely an issue in clinical anesthesia.

Clinical Use

It is a widespread practice in the United States for anesthesia providers to administer a dose of fentanyl to patients, either just before or just after their entry into an operating room. It would seem that there is a universal presumption that every surgical patient has "an acute fentanyl deficiency" that must be treated promptly. In most cases, a better choice would be meperidine if the anesthetic and operation are projected to last more than 90 min. The reasons for this are several. First, the onset of action of meperidine is sufficiently close to that of fentanyl (5 min vs. 1–2 min) that it will provide sedation and analgesia in a timely manner. Second, it will suppress the cough reflex and attenuate the cardiovascular responses to tracheal intubation similar to fentanyl. Meperidine 0.3–0.4 mg/kg (20–30 mg in adults) will have the same induction effect as fentanyl (50–100 µg). It just has to be given a few minutes earlier than fentanyl because it is not quite as lipid soluble. Third, it is an excellent opiate, about one-tenth as potent as morphine, with alpha 2 agonist and local anesthetic properties [8] thereby providing multimodal analgesia during surgery. Presuming a near MAC level of anesthesia with sevoflurane, isoflurane, or desflurane, alone or in combination with nitrous oxide, the addition of meperidine will raise the MAC level to 1.2–1.4 and provide the necessary analgesia for the operation to proceed smoothly. A heart rate elevated above the resting baseline is an indication that more meperidine is needed. The usual incremental doses of meperidine are 20–30 mg in adults, and the peak effect of each dose will occur within about 10 min. When adequate analgesia has been achieved, the heart rate will return to baseline. An elevated heart rate is an indication that not enough meperidine has been given or that the patient is hypovolemic and needs intravenous fluid (see Addendum for case examples).

A curious event occurs when patients receive meperidine in combination with nitrous oxide 50–70 %. Some type of interaction occurs between the two drugs causing a decrease in heart rate, usually to a rate of 50–60 bpm. This only occurs if the total dose of meperidine is sufficient to provide adequate analgesia, and the patient is not hypovolemic. This interaction is unique to the meperidine–N_2O combination; it does not occur with meperidine and volatile anesthetics (sevoflurane, isoflurane). Although a common occurrence, this interaction in man has never been reported in the literature and the mechanism is unknown.

The total dose of meperidine administered will depend on several factors including dose of volatile or other agents being administered, age and size of patient, whether patient is tolerant to opiates because of prior use, and type and duration of surgery. As a general guide, it is ideal to administer from 2 to 3 mg/kg meperidine in divided doses over the course of a 90–180 min surgery. At these total dose levels, patients will emerge from general anesthesia promptly, have satisfactory respiratory function, and respond appropriately to questions or commands. A really nice feature is that the patients will not shiver on awakening or in the recovery room. If the total dose is 1 mg/kg or less, the patient will generally not have any appreciable level of analgesia upon emergence from anesthesia. However, this is not a serious issue since additional doses of meperidine can be administered after emergence, and each dose will provide a level of analgesia within 5 min. There is one caveat with the use of meperidine. All administration of meperidine should be terminated 1 h before the end of surgery. If any is administered in the last hour, it will make the patient more somnolent and delay removal of the endotracheal tube.

If asked if they are in pain, patients will often say yes, but will not complain of pain. If a patient does complain of pain, a 20–30 mg dose of meperidine intravenously will usually resolve the problem temporarily. Concomitant with giving a temporizing dose of meperidine, one may administer a therapeutic dose of morphine or dihydromorphone. By the time the morphine drugs are producing their pharmacological effects, the meperidine will be waning, so there is minimal concern about opioid overdose. In effect, meperidine is a good transitional analgesic in the postoperative period.

Like virtually all other opioid narcotics, meperidine will cause nausea and vomiting in some patients. What comparative studies exist suggest that the incidence of nausea and vomiting is equal to or greater with meperidine than with other opiates, but the differences are relatively small. Further, what studies exist are not compelling enough to select one opiate over another based on the likelihood that one can avoid nausea and vomiting. Administration of ondansetron 4 mg, metoclopramide 10 mg and dexamethasone 5–10 mg prior to emergence from anesthesia will almost always completely prevent early postoperative nausea and vomiting from meperidine administered intraoperatively. When patients are switched postoperatively to other opiate narcotics, it is very likely that the antiemetics cited above will need to be continued.

Summary

Meperidine has been denigrated in many medical and pharmacological publications for good reasons when used to manage most types of pain [5, 6], but it still has an important and valuable place in clinical anesthesia. As an intravenous analgesic in the operating room, there is no better drug for operations lasting more than 90 min. The drug is dispensed in 100 mg vials or ampules, which is best diluted to 10 mg/mL with sterile water or saline in a 10 mL syringe. The initial and subsequent doses are easy to remember: adult 20–30 mg; 10-year-old 10 mg; 5-year-old 5 mg. At a stable level of inhalation or intravenous anesthesia, meperidine tells the anesthesia provider when more should be given. Clinical signs of increased heart rate and blood pressure indicate the need for additional meperidine. With each dose the vital signs will return to baseline, and with subsequent doses, the intervals before needing another dose will become more prolonged. What could be easier!! Try to administer at least 2 mg/kg (and more if the operation is extremely painful), and do not give any the last hour of the operation. Once awake, it is a useful transitional drug to relieve pain while establishing a blood level of a more effective, long-term analgesic such as dihydromorphone. It is superior to fentanyl or its derivatives in many preoperative, operative, and immediate postoperative situations because of its rapid onset, effective multimodal analgesic profile, and avoidance of sudden apnea when standard doses are used.

Addendum

Case 1

A 26 year old, 96 kg man was admitted to the emergency room of a hospital following an accident on a freeway in which his motorcycle was broadsided by an automobile. His major injuries were a fractured right femur and open right tibia-fibula fractures. There were multiple minor lacerations of the arms and legs but no head or internal injuries. He denied eating before the early morning accident. An intravenous catheter was inserted and he was give dihydromorphone 2.5 mg in divided doses for pain relief. After complete evaluation, he was taken to the operating room for orthopedic repair of both injuries.

His preoperative vital signs were blood pressure 136/77 mmHg, pulse 92 b/min, respiration 12/min, EKG normal sinus rhythm, and oxygen saturation 99 % breathing room air. Because of his fractures, regional anesthesia was out of the question. After preoxygenation, general anesthesia was induced with meperidine 30 mg, propofol 60 mg, rocuronium 100 mg, sevoflurane 1 % and oxygen. With cricoid pressure, gentle, controlled ventilation was started and continued until full paralysis occurred. Standard endotracheal intubation was accomplished and mechanical ventilation initiated. After tracheal intubation his blood pressure increased to

144/87 mmHg and pulse to 98 b/min so an additional dose of meperidine 20 mg was administered. Nitrous oxide 60 % was started and the sevoflurane concentration was decreased to 0.6 %.

Over the next hour of surgery he received meperidine 120 mg in 20 mg increments. The blood pressure stabilized at 128/68 mmHg and pulse at 62 b/min. Over the next 3½h he received additional meperidine 80 mg in 20 mg increments, the indication for each dose being an increase in heart rate to >70 b/min. With each dose the heart rate returned to the low 60 range within 5 min, and the maximum change occurred within 10 min. As well, the time intervals between meperidine doses became progressively longer. Serial hematocrit values were followed and maintained >30 % with transfusion of packed red blood cells. The total dose of meperidine in the 4½h case was 250 mg or 2.6 mg/kg, none being given the last hour of the operation. Near the end of surgery, the blood pressure and pulse increased, and the dose of sevoflurane was increased to 1.5 %. About 30 min before the anticipated end of surgery, the nitrous oxide was rapidly eliminated by high flow oxygen, keeping the sevoflurane at the same concentration. When the inspired oxygen concentration reached 80 %, the ventilator was turned off. With no ventilation, the patient's arterial carbon dioxide level increased, and at an end tidal value of 46 mmHg, spontaneous ventilation ensued. The sevoflurane administration was stopped and within a few minutes the patient started reacting to the endotracheal tube. With intact airway reflexes the endotracheal tube was removed. The patient coughed and was asked to take a deep breath, which he did. He lay quietly with his eyes closed, but when asked if he has pain, he said yes. He was given meperidine 20 mg and transported to the recovery room breathing oxygen from a transport mask. Having been given the antiemetics noted in the text, he denied any nausea. Orders were left for him to receive dihydromorphone 0.3 mg q30 min for pain. Postoperatively he did well and was delighted with his anesthetic care.

Case 2

A 66-year-old 58 kg woman was admitted to hospital with a diagnosis of a tumor of the mandible, which extended into soft tissue on the right side of her neck. Her airway was not compromised by the tumor. She had no other medical issues. In the holding area prior to surgery she was given midazolam 2 mg intravenously. On arrival in the operating room she was given meperidine 20 mg. After preoxygenation, anesthesia was induced with propofol 40 mg and sevoflurane 1 %. Once it was established that controlled ventilation was easily accomplished, rocuronium 50 mg was administered. An LMA # 3 was inserted and the patient was placed on controlled ventilation. With the operator's hands now freed up, cocaine 4 % pledgets were placed in the left nostril. Anticipating a circulatory response to tracheal intubation, another 20 mg meperidine was administered. A fiberoptic scope was inserted into the left nostril and when it reached the oropharynx, the LMA was removed. The scope was advanced into the larynx followed by a 6.0 nasotracheal tube.

The surgery lasted 7.5 h and consisted of removal of the right mandible and a right neck dissection, construction of a new mandible using a fibular graft, and vascularization of a soft tissue graft from the abdomen to the neck. During this time the patient received meperidine in 20 mg increments at ever more prolonged intervals, for a total dose of 160 mg or about 2.8 mg/kg. Nitrous oxide 60 % and sevoflurane 0.6 % were also administered. Heart rate remained in the low 60-b/min range, increasing only when additional meperidine was needed. No meperidine was administered the last 90 min of the surgery. Once final closure was underway, the nitrous oxide was rapidly eliminated and the sevoflurane concentration increased to 1.2 %. Controlled ventilation was stopped when the inspired oxygen concentration in the circuit reached 80 %. Spontaneous ventilation ensued when the end tidal carbon dioxide concentration reached 52 mmHg. The inspired sevoflurane concentration was decreased and the end tidal CO_2 value gradually decreased to 46 %. About 6 min after stopping the sevoflurane, the patient opened her eyes and responded to the command to take a deep breath. When asked whether she was in pain she shook her head no. She was taken to the recovery room breathing oxygen via the nasotracheal tube. When she was fully awake, the nasotracheal tube was removed. She was maintained postoperatively for a day on dihydromorphone 0.1–0.2 mg for pain relief. The remainder of her recovery was uneventful.

These two cases are typical examples of the successful use of meperidine in surgical anesthesia. They demonstrate the usual size and timing of the doses, the indications for its administration, and the responses to each dose. Because of its rapid onset and reasonable duration of action, and the fact that vital signs indicate when additional doses are needed make it a very easy, safe and reliable opiate for use in surgical anesthesia expected to last more than 60–90 min.

References

1. Eisleb O, Schaumann O. Dolantin, ein neuartiges spasmolytikum und analgetikum (chemisches und pharmakologisches). Dtsch Med Wschr. 1939;65:967–8.
2. Schaumann O. Uber eine neue klasse von verbindungen mit spasmolytischer und zentral analgrtischer wirksamkeit unter besonderer berucksichtigung des 1-methyl-4phenyl-piperidin-4-carbonsaure-athylesters (dolantin). Archiv f Experiment Path u Pharmakol. 1940;196:109–36.
3. Rovenstine EA, Batterman RC. The utility of Demerol as a substitute for the opiates in preanesthetic medication. Anesthesiology. 1943;4:126–34.
4. Batterman RC, Himmelsbach CK. Demerol—a new synthetic analgesic. JAMA. 1943;122:222–6.
5. Latta KS, Ginsberg B, Barkin RL. Meperidine: a critical review. Am J Ther. 2002;9:53–68.
6. Dobyns JB. Anesthesia for the patient with asthma. Curr Rev Clin Anesth. 2015;35:229–40.
7. Takada K, Clark DJ, Davies MF, Tonner PH, Krause TK, Bertaccini E, Maze M. Meperidine exerts agonist activity at the alpha (2B)-adrenoceptor subtype. Anesthesiology. 2002;96:1420–6.
8. Jaffe RA, Rowe MA. A comparison of the local anesthetic effects of meperidine, fentanyl, and sufentanil on dorsal root axons. Anesth Analg. 1996;83:776–81.

Chapter 11
Sevoflurane: The Best Volatile Anesthetic Ever Developed

Introduction

Over the past 50 years there have been three gas and 13 volatile anesthetic agents made available for clinical use.

Inhalation anesthetics used over last 50 years
Nitrous oxide*
Ethylene
Cyclopropane
Diethyl ether
Chloroform
Ethyl chloride
Divinyl ether (Vinethene)
Ethyl vinyl ether (Vinamar)
Trichlorethylene (Trilene)
Fluroxene
Halothane (Fluothane)*
Methoxyflurane (Penthrane)
Enflurane
Isoflurane (Forane)*
Sevoflurane (Ultane)*
Desflurane (Suprane)*

Trade name given in parentheses
*Drugs still available for clinical use

Of the three gas anesthetics only nitrous oxide continues to be used widely, primarily because of its effectiveness, ease of administration, and low cost. Among the 13 other agents, based on both scientific data from the literature and extensive,

© Springer International Publishing Switzerland 2017
C.P. Larson Jr., R.A. Jaffe, *Practical Anesthetic Management*,
DOI 10.1007/978-3-319-42866-6_11

personal clinical experience with all 13 that **sevoflurane is the best volatile anesthetic ever developed**. What follows will be a brief history of the drug, and consideration of those attributes that make is such a valuable anesthetic.

Historical Development

The development of sevoflurane is an unusual and truly remarkable story. In the late 1960s, four investigators at Travenol Laboratories in Morton Grove, Illinois began evaluating the inhalation anesthetic properties of a group of halogenated methyl isopropyl ethers. Their hope was to find an inhalation anesthetic that would be superior to halothane, which dominated the market at that time [1]. They investigated a number of compounds, the most promising being fluromethyl 2,2,2-trifluoro-1-[trifluoromethyl] ethyl (Fig. 11.1), which was given the name sevoflurane. Subsequent investigators Thomas Cook, Richard Mazze and Michael Halsey performed a variety of studies in mice, rats and dogs, administering sevoflurane for brief or prolonged periods and with single or multiple exposures without observing any serious sequellae [2]. However, two features about the drug emerged that were of concern. The first was that sevoflurane underwent biotransformation, which resulted in increases in inorganic fluoride ions in 24-h urine samples. The urinary inorganic fluoride levels were higher in mice given sevoflurane than those given halothane or isoflurane, but far below levels produced by methoxyflurane. The second concern was the fact that sevoflurane reacted with soda lime to form two substances identified by mass spectroscopy as compounds A and B.

Despite the favorable findings in the original report by Wallin et al. [1], there was very little interest in studying this anesthetic further, probably for three reasons. First, there was a longstanding, hallowed dictum in anesthesiology, which decried the development or use of any anesthetic that reacted with soda lime, regardless of what the derived product(s) might be. This tenet was based on prior experience with trichloroethylene, which decomposed to phosgene, hydrochloric acid, and carbon monoxide when exposed to warm soda lime for several hours. Clinical reports of cranial nerve palsies, particularly the fifth cranial nerve terminated its use soon after halothane became available. The second reason relates to the fact that Mazze and colleagues had just published their findings with methoxyflurane, which showed a

Fig. 11.1 Chemical
structure of sevoflurane

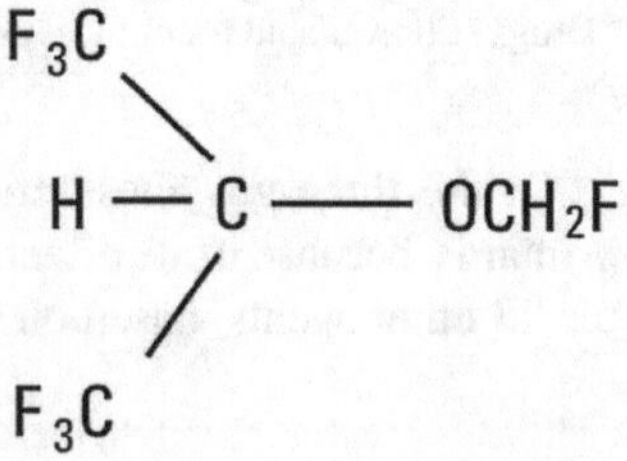

$$F_3C$$
$$\diagdown$$
$$H - C \longrightarrow OCH_2F$$
$$\diagup$$
$$F_3C$$

dose-related nephrotoxicity in rats owing to its biotransformation to inorganic fluoride ions. While preliminary studies indicated that inorganic fluoride ion levels with sevoflurane were nowhere near as high or as prolonged as with methoxyflurane, neither halothane nor isoflurane, a newly developed volatile anesthetic at that time, caused any appreciable increase in serum or urinary fluoride levels. And third, since halothane remained a suitable drug for inhalation induction anesthesia, and isoflurane underwent less biotransformation than sevoflurane (1 vs. 3%), and was a suitable maintenance agent, there was little incentive to investigate sevoflurane further.

However, Duncan Holaday and Burnell Brown were attracted to sevoflurane because of its pleasant smell, low blood-gas solubility (0.65), and hence rapid induction and recovery, and lack of cardiac arrhythmias when epinephrine is administered. In 1981 Holaday and Smith published a phase-1 study of the clinical characteristics and biotransformation of sevoflurane in six healthy volunteers exposed to 2–3% for 1 h [3]. They observed stable respiratory and cardiovascular function, rapid induction and emergence with no aberrant behavior (coughing, shivering, retching, laryngospasm), limited biotransformation (about 3% of the administered drug), and no toxic effects. Inorganic serum fluoride levels averaged 22 μmol/l, well below the values seen with methoxyflurane, and returned to normal values within 24 h after termination of the anesthetic. Their conclusion was that phase-2 and phase-3 clinical trials should commence. This didn't happen. For the next 10 years no further clinical studies of sevoflurane were conducted. It was not until 1991 that Yasuda et al. published a study in which they compared the kinetics of sevoflurane and isoflurane in man [4]. In fact, Brown and Frink wrote an editorial in 1992 asking "Whatever happened to sevoflurane?" What happened was that the drug got lost in the shuffle as interest became directed toward the development of better intravenous anesthetics [5]. Baxter Travenol sold sevoflurane to the British Oxygen Corporation, which reorganized and changed its name to Ohmeda. Ohmeda, knowing that desflurane was in the final developmental stages sold sevoflurane to Mariushi, a Japanese pharmaceutical company. The drug was licensed in Japan and subsequently administered to several million Japanese without any apparent, serious complications. Based on this favorable experience, Mariushi Pharmaceuticals contracted with Abbott Laboratories to facilitate approval of the drug by the FDA, and subsequent distribution in the United States. Many phase 2 and 3 studies were done, and the drug was approved by the FDA in 1994, and became widely available in the United States in 1995.

Pharmacological Properties of Sevoflurane

Solubility

What are the special pharmacological characteristics of sevoflurane that make it the most valuable volatile anesthetic ever developed? There are several. Most important among these is its **low blood-gas partition coefficient of 0.65**.

Favorable characteristics of Sevoflurane
Low blood-gas solubility coefficient (0.65)
Rapid induction and recovery
Potent, can be used with oxygen only
Pleasant, non-irritating smell
Minimal or no stimulation of airway reflexes
Laryngospasm during induction or emergence uncommon
Suitable for inhalation induction in all ages
Standard, agent-specific vaporizer used
Cardiovascular and respiratory functions maintained
Protects heart from ischemia
Compatible with epinephrine and norepinephrine

This means that for every sevoflurane molecule in the blood phase, there are nearly two molecules in the gas phase. As a result **both induction and emergence from sevoflurane anesthesia are rapid.** Because sevoflurane has a slightly higher blood-gas partition coefficient than nitrous oxide (0.65 vs. 0.47), clinicians often discontinue sevoflurane near the conclusion of an anesthetic, but continue with nitrous oxide administration, expecting that with this technique the patient will emerge from anesthesia faster. While possibly true, this is a misguided practice for several reasons. First, the difference in emergence time between the two drugs is trivial (<5 min), and differences in recovery responses among patients are greater than the solubility difference between the two anesthetics. Second, it is much easier and safer to have a patient transition from controlled ventilation to spontaneous breathing with the lungs full of oxygen than with lungs containing nitrous oxide 50–60 %. Provided the anesthesiologist avoids airway obstruction via an endotracheal tube or LMA, substantial loss of lung volume from abdominal or thoracic compression, or inadequate reversal of neuromuscular blockade, a patient can go for a prolonged period without breathing and not sustain any degree of oxygen desaturation when the lungs are filled with oxygen-sevoflurane. The same is not true when the lungs contain nitrous oxide 50–60 %. When the lungs contain a substantial concentration of nitrous oxide, the anesthesia provider must watch the pulse oximeter closely, and ventilate the lungs regularly to avoid oxygen desaturation. This requirement for periodic ventilation delays return of spontaneous ventilation because it slows the rate of carbon dioxide accumulation and hence the stimulus to breathe. Thirdly, if patients should inadvertently cough or buck on an endotracheal tube or LMA during the transition from controlled to spontaneous ventilation, the severity of oxygen desaturation is worse when the lungs contain nitrous oxide than when they contain sevoflurane-oxygen. And lastly, if a patient should become unacceptably light during the terminal phases of an operation, the anesthesia provider can increase the sevoflurane concentration and total oxygen flow, and the level of anesthesia will very rapidly deepen to an acceptable level. The reasons that this works so quickly are twofold. First, the patient already has substantial venous and tissue concentrations of sevoflurane, so very little must to be added to the alveolar, arterial blood and brain concentrations to achieve a deeper plane of anesthesia. And second, the low solubility coefficient makes the uptake of sevoflurane rapid. The same is not true when nitrous oxide is used. Given its lower potency, one cannot increase the nitrous oxide concentration safely to a level that will resolve the need for more anesthesia, so an intravenous drug (e.g. propofol, thiopental, lidocaine) must be administered. Depending upon the dose administered, and other prevailing factors, the patient may become apneic necessitating controlled ventilation for a time.

Patient safety is greatly enhanced by discontinuing nitrous oxide rather than sevoflurane near the conclusion of a nitrous oxide-sevoflurane anesthetic.

In contrast to human tissues, sevoflurane is soluble in soda lime, and five times more soluble in baralyme, with the solubility increasing in both absorbents as absorbent temperature increases. However, it has been shown that the absorption of sevoflurane in soda lime has minimal effects on the clinical characteristics of the drug.

Potency

Sevoflurane is also a potent drug, having MAC values averaging about 2% in middle-aged adults, up to 3% in young children, and about 1.5% in those 70 years and above. The addition of nitrous oxide, 60% decreases the MAC of sevoflurane by about 50% [6]. Sevoflurane is a complete inhalation anesthetic in that it will produce amnesia, analgesia and elimination of unwanted reflexes at concentrations of 2–4%, thus allowing for the use of high concentrations of oxygen (>95%) if indicated. Sevoflurane-oxygen anesthesia may be useful for patients undergoing intrathoracic or intra-abdominal operations, or those who have relatively severe chronic obstructive lung disease. Sevoflurane-oxygen anesthesia may also be useful for patients who are undergoing spine surgery with somatosensory evoked potential (SSEP) monitoring is planned. Sevoflurane at 2–3% concentrations interferes less with SSEP tracings than does nitrous oxide-sevoflurane anesthesia. However sevoflurane may also be used in combination with nitrous oxide in many operative procedures, thereby decreasing its utilization rate by 50–60% at any total gas flow rate. A standard, calibrated, agent-specific vaporizer is used to vaporize the agent and deliver it to the anesthetic circuit.

Optimum Airway Properties

Sevoflurane has a pleasant, non-irritating aroma, which allows for inhalation inductions in patients of all ages, not just infants and children as originally suggested. It is an excellent drug for inhalation induction in adult patients who are afraid of needle sticks, or those who are devoid of obvious veins for intravenous access while awake (e.g.: burn patients, the morbidly obese, or patients on prolonged treatment with chemotherapeutic agents). One of several induction techniques may be used. One can introduce the drug gradually using either just oxygen or nitrous oxide-oxygen as carrier gases, or have the patient take 4–5 deep breaths of a high concentration (up to 8%) with or without preloading the anesthetic circuit. With either technique amnesia occurs within 1 min, and surgical levels of anesthesia within 5–10 min. Also, there is little or no airway irritability or stimulation of airway reflexes with rapid inhalation induction with sevoflurane. Laryngospasm rarely occurs during induction even when sevoflurane is administered in high or rapidly increasing concentrations. Likewise, compared with other inhaled anesthetics, laryngospasm is also rare during emergence from sevoflurane anesthesia. This is an important feature of sevoflurane, since laryngospasm delays both induction and recovery, and if not promptly resolved may cause negative pressure pulmonary edema.

Its low blood-gas solubility, potency, pleasant odor and lack of airway irritability make sevoflurane an excellent agent for inhalation inductions in patients of all ages.

Circulatory Effects

Many clinical studies of sevoflurane have been published in recent years that support and amplify on the earlier pharmacological studies. In general they show that the circulatory effects are no worse than, and in some cases better than for other inhalation agents. In healthy patients, sevoflurane produces a dose-dependent decrease in blood pressure primarily as a result of a decrease in systemic vascular resistance (afterload reduction), with either no change or a slight decrease in heart rate. At MAC the decreases in blood pressure are modest, are no greater than those seen with other inhalation anesthetics, and are rapidly reversed by decreasing the inspired concentration. At 2 MAC the decreases in blood pressure are greater than at MAC, and are due to both vascular dilatation and myocardial depression. These decreases are mitigated somewhat by increases in heart rate. One of the marvelous advantages of sevoflurane is its safety profile when administered gradually as an inhalation induction either alone or following a minimal dose of an intravenous induction agent to patients who are hypovolemic from hemorrhage or uncontrolled hypertension, or who have severe cardiovascular disease. Also, some seemingly healthy patients occasionally have an unexpectedly profound adverse cardiovascular response to standard doses of intravenous and inhalation drugs. Decreasing the inspired concentration or terminating administration when the agent is sevoflurane as compared to isoflurane or halothane much more readily reverses hypotension that occurs in these kinds of patients.

Sevoflurane does not stimulate catecholamine output, nor does it predispose the heart to arrhythmias when catecholamines are administered for control of surgical bleeding. It has been shown that sevoflurane may prolong the Q–T interval on the electrocardiogram, and it has been suggested that it should be administered cautiously in the rare patient whose Q–T interval is abnormally prolonged. In one study, infants under 6 months of age given a sevoflurane anesthetic developed a prolonged

Q–T interval compared to those given a halothane anesthetic, and the prolongation lasted more than 1 h after termination of the anesthetic [7]. However, prolongation of the Q–T interval occurs with other anesthetic and nonanesthetic drugs, and there is no evidence to date in infants or adults that it is of any clinical significance.

Sevoflurane may cause prolongation of the Q–T interval in some patients, but its clinical significance remains unknown.

Recent studies in animals and man suggest that sevoflurane, like other volatile anesthetics protects the heart from ischemia, although the exact mechanism for this cardioprotective effect is not clear. For example, several investigators have shown that a brief exposure to sevoflurane protects the isolated rat or guinea pig heart model from ischemia-reperfusion injury, perhaps by enhancing mitochondrial channel opening (activating adenosine triphosphate-regulated potassium [K_{ATP}] channels, or suppressing mitochondrial respiratory function [8]. A recent study in high-risk patients who were undergoing coronary artery bypass surgery suggested that sevoflurane anesthesia preserved left ventricular function operatively and postoperatively better than propofol [9]. Sevoflurane is known to cause coronary vasodilatation, and as a result may increase blood flow retrograde via collateral coronary vessels to potentially ischemic myocardium.

Respiratory Effects

For the most part, the respiratory effects of sevoflurane are not appreciably different from those for other anesthetic drugs. Sevoflurane decreases tidal volume in a dose-dependent manner without appreciable change in respiratory frequency. As a result, end tidal and arterial CO_2 values increase as depth of anesthesia increases. Ventilatory responses to a carbon dioxide challenge decrease with increasing depth of anesthesia, as would be expected. Of course, these effects are mitigated by surgical stimulation. Sevoflurane, like other volatile anesthetics, is a bronchodilator. The most important difference between sevoflurane and other volatile anesthetics is the fact that sevoflurane does not cause airway irritability. As a result it is the best agent that we have for inducing anesthesia by inhalation in infants, children, and adults. Finally, sevoflurane like other volatile anesthetics has minimal effect on the normal hypoxic pulmonary vasoconstriction response, as evidenced by the finding that oxygenation is well maintained during one-lung ventilation.

Neuroanesthesia Effects

Although there is some variability in results among clinical studies, the predominant finding is that sevoflurane causes a dose-dependent increase in both total and regional cerebral blood. Cerebral oxygen consumption is decreased by a commensurate amount so that oxygen delivery exceeds oxygen demand. The increase in

CBF and consequently cerebral blood volume results in an increase in intracranial pressure (ICP) [10]. However, the increase in ICP that is undesirable in patients with brain tumors or other space-occupying lesions can by prevented or corrected by hyperventilation and lowering of arterial CO_2 or by administering drugs such as propofol or thiopental intravenously.

Sevoflurane-oxygen anesthesia at concentrations of MAC or less, supplemented with opiates to achieve an adequate level of anesthesia is a technique that has little adverse effects on somatosensory evoked potentials (SSEP's). Avoidance of nitrous oxide enhances SSEP monitoring during sevoflurane anesthesia.

Renal Effects

One of the major concerns regarding the use of sevoflurane is the fact that about 5 % of the inhaled drug is metabolized in the liver to inorganic fluoride ions, which are then excreted via the kidneys. When the kidneys are exposed to a high concentration of inorganic fluoride ions for a prolonged period, nephrotoxicity as evidenced by high output renal failure develops. However, many studies in patients with normal renal function, and several studies in patients with stable renal insufficiency have shown that sevoflurane does not cause any renal abnormalities not seen with equal frequency with isoflurane [11]. Even though sevoflurane is associated with higher levels of serum inorganic fluoride than isoflurane, the levels are not either high enough or sustained for a long enough period of time to cause nephrotoxicity. This finding is true even when total gas flows are 1 L/min or less.

The second issue with sevoflurane is its reaction with soda lime to form Compound A. The amount of Compound A formed is greater the lower the fresh gas flow, the dryer and hotter the carbon dioxide absorbent, the higher the sevoflurane concentration, and the longer the duration of exposure of sevoflurane to the absorbent. Compound A at 50 ppm has been shown to cause cortical necrosis in the rat kidney. Similar results have not been observed in other animal species including the dog, cat, monkey, or in humans. In one study, patients with stable renal insufficiency exposed to >3 h of sevoflurane at 0.8–2.5 vol.% and a total gas flow of <1 L/min showed an average Compound A concentration in the anesthetic circuit of 13 ppm, and a maximum concentration of 19 ppm. No patient showed any abnormality postoperatively in either serum creatinine or BUN. Gentz and Malan reviewed the literature and concluded that "Compound A values must exceed 150 ppm/h to produce any changes in markers of renal function, and whatever changes do occur are mild and always reversible." They labeled the whole issue "a storm in a teacup" [12].

Sevoflurane is safe to administer to patients with impaired renal function or those undergoing renal transplantation as well as healthy patients even at total gas flow rates of 1 L/min.

Although Abbott Laboratories recommends that sevoflurane exposure should not exceed 2 MAC-hours at flow rates of 1–2 L/min, there is no body of scientific evidence in patients to support that recommendation.

Hepatic Effects

Animal studies indicate that sevoflurane has very little effect on hepatic blood flow. Likewise, although sevoflurane undergoes some (about 3 %) metabolism in the liver, there is no convincing evidence documenting that the metabolic products are hepatotoxic. Sevoflurane, unlike other volatile anesthetics does not result in the formation of hepatotoxic fluoroacetylated antibodies. Existing data would support the conclusion that sevoflurane is perfectly safe to use in patients with hepatic disease or impairment.

Adverse Effects of Sevoflurane

Malignant Hyperthermia

While sevoflurane is the best volatile anesthetic ever developed, it is certainly not perfect. The adverse side effects are few in number, but important to remember.

Unfavorable characteristics of Sevoflurane
Triggering agent for malignant hyperthermia
Emergence dysphoria in children
Nausea/vomiting
Seizures
Carbon monoxide production
Fire in anesthesia circuit

Certainly the most important adverse effect of sevoflurane is one that it shares with all of the other volatile anesthetics, namely its ability to precipitate malignant hyperthermia (MH) in susceptible patients. While a very rare event, it is one of which anesthesia providers must be cognizant when administering the drug. What isn't known is whether MH, if detected early in patients is less severe or more readily reversible than when caused by isoflurane or halothane because of sevoflurane's much lower solubility, and hence much faster excretion rate.

Emergence Dysphoria

A second area of concern is the dysphoria or agitation observed in infants and children during emergence from sevoflurane anesthesia. The incidence of agitation seems to be in the 15–20 % range, with the higher incidence being in the younger age groups. It has been shown not to be due entirely to postoperative pain, since it occurs in infants and children who undergo diagnostic or therapeutic radiological procedures where no pain is involved. While the agitation is relatively short lived (usually >30 min), it is troublesome for recovery room nurses, and of concern to parents who may observe the behavior. A variety of agents have been suggested including fentanyl and midazolam to prevent or lessen the agitation. One group showed that clonidine 4 μg/kg given orally as a premedicant prevented the postoperative agitation in children 2–11 years of age who underwent minor surgery under sevoflurane anesthesia [13].

Nausea/Vomiting

About 25 % of patients receiving sevoflurane experience nausea with or without vomiting in the early postoperative period (PONV). This incidence is considerably lower than that reported in patients given desflurane (60–70 %). There are several methods to avoid or resolve PONV. For patients who have a prior history of PONV following anesthesia, one can avoid nitrous oxide which may exacerbate the likelihood of PONV, and/or administer dolasetron 10 mg, droperidol 0.625 mg, metaclopromide 10 mg, dexamethasone 5 mg, or a subhypnotic dose of propofol 0.5 mg/kg near the termination of anesthesia. Many choose to administer both a dopamine (droperidol, metaclopromide) and serotonin (dolasetron, odansetron) receptor antagonist, since these are believed to be the two major mechanisms for PONV. If the history is one of severe PONV, one can add dexamethasone to the prescription. This combination of drugs also works well as rescue medication, and must be continued postoperatively for as long as the patient is receiving opiate analgesics. We do not use propofol because it prolongs the emergence phase of anesthesia, and has not been shown to be superior to the combination therapy noted above.

Seizures

Motor activity resembling a seizure has been reported in both adults and children during induction or emergence from sevoflurane anesthesia. In most cases it was difficult for the observers to distinguish clinically between a seizure and motor activity associated with agitation or excitement. In one study in children, agitation during induction was not associated with any seizure-like electroencephalographic patterns [14]. True focal or grand mal seizures are rare, and when they have occurred, they have not resulted in any documented neurological sequellae.

Carbon Monoxide Production

Carbon monoxide (CO) production from the flow of sevoflurane through soda lime has been reported, but the concentrations recorded are miniscule compared to the values reported for desflurane or isoflurane. The highest CO concentrations were observed in the laboratory when dry (desiccated) soda lime, low flows (<2 L/min), and high concentration of sevoflurane (5 %) were used. This combination of events rarely occurs in the clinical setting, and hence the rarity of clinical reports of CO poisoning in humans.

Fire in the Anesthesia Circuit

Abbott Laboratories sent a letter to all anesthesia personnel alerting them of rare, isolated reports of fire or extreme heat in anesthesia circuits when sevoflurane is administered through dry soda lime. Neither the incidence nor severity of the heat or fire was detailed in the letter. Abbott implied that the major cause was dry soda lime, and recommended that gas flows be terminated at the conclusion of anesthesia, and that circuit canisters be loaded with fresh soda lime when anesthesia machines have been unused for extended periods. They also suggested that signs of a problem include a soda lime canister that is unusually hot to touch, and a growing disparity between the sevoflurane vaporizer setting (higher) and the inspired gas concentration (lower). Current evidence certainly suggests that dry (desiccated) soda lime is the major culprit behind excessive Compound A, carbon monoxide production, and excessive heat and fires in the anesthesia circuit. It would seem that these rare events could be made virtually nonexistent by refreshing soda lime canisters whenever there is any question about their viability.

Summary

Without question, sevoflurane is the best volatile anesthetic ever developed. Its major assets are its potency, low solubility, lack of airway irritation, ease of administration, rapid induction and recovery, ease of reversal if hypotension or other adverse events occur, myocardial protection from ischemia, and low incidence of PONV compared to other volatile agents. Nephrotoxicity from Compound A or fluoride ions is a nonentity in both healthy patients and those with renal impairment. The other adverse effects of sevoflurane are rare, and except for malignant hyperthermia can be avoided by utilization of fresh soda lime.

References

1. Wallin RF, Regan BM, Napoli MD, Stern IJ. Sevoflurane: a new inhalational anesthetic agent. Anesth Analg. 1975;54:758–66.
2. Cook TL, Beppu WJ, Hitt BA, Kosek JC, Mazze RI. Renal effects and metabolism of sevoflurane in Fischer 344 rats: an in-vivo and in vitro comparison with methoxyflurane. Anesthesiology. 1975;43:70–7.

3. Holaday DA, Smith FR. Clinical characteristics and biotransformation of sevoflurane in healthy human volunteers. Anesthesiology. 1981;54:100–6.
4. Yasuda N, Lockhart SH, Eger EI, Weiskopf RB, Liu J, Laster M, Taheri S, Peterson NA. Comparison of kinetics of sevoflurane and isoflurane in humans. Anesth Analg. 1991;72:316–24.
5. Brown BR, Frink EJ. Whatever happened to sevoflurane? Can J Anaesth. 1992;39:207–9.
6. Fragen RJ, Dunn KL. The minimum alveolar concentration (MAC) of sevoflurane with and without nitrous oxide in elderly versus young adults. J Clin Anesth. 1996;8:352–6.
7. Loeckinger A, Kleinsasser A, Maier S, Furtner B, Keller C, Kuehbacher G, Lindner KH. Sustained prolongation of the QTc interval after anesthesia with sevoflurane in infants during the first 6 months of life. Anesthesiology. 2003;98:639–42.
8. Varadarajan SG, An J, Novalija E, Stowe DF. Sevoflurane before or after ischemia improves contractile and metabolic function while reducing myoplasmic Ca^{2+} loading in intact hearts. Anesthesiology. 2002;96:125–33.
9. DeHert SG, tenBroecke PW, Mertens E, Van Sommeren EW, DeBlier IG, Stockman BA, Rodrigus IE. Sevoflurane but not propofol preserves myocardial function in coronary surgery patients. Anesthesiology. 2002;97:42–9.
10. Petersen KD, Landsfeldt U, Cold GE, Petersen CB, Mau S, Hauerberg J, Holst P, Olsen KS. Intracranial pressure and cerebral hemodynamic in patients with cerebral tumors. Anesthesiology. 2003;98:329–36.
11. Conzen PF, Kharasch ED, Czerner SFA, Atru AA, Reichle FM, Michalowski P, Rooke GA, Weiss BM, Ebert TJ. Low-flow sevoflurane compared with low-flow isoflurane anesthesia in patients with stable renal insufficiency. Anesthesiology. 2002;97:578–84.
12. Gentz BA, Malan Jr TP. Renal toxicity with sevoflurane. A storm in a teacup? Drugs. 2001;61:2155–62.
13. Mikawa K, Nishina K, Shiga M. Prevention of sevoflurane-induced agitation with oral clonidine premedication. Anesth Analg. 2002;94:1675–6.
14. Constant I, Dubois MC, Piat V, Moutard ML, McCue M, Murat I. Changes in electroencephalogram and autonomic cardiovascular activity during induction of anesthesia with sevoflurane compared with halothane in children. Anesthesiology. 1999;91:1604–15.

Chapter 12
The Bariatric Challenge

Introduction

Obesity is a major health hazard both nationally and internationally for three reasons. First, although there are not reliable statistical data documenting the rate of increase in obesity in the Unites States, both the lay and medical press state with conviction that the number of people moving into the obese category is alarming (Fig. 12.1). Second, obesity is a disease, and as such alters the normal physiologic functions of the body. And third, obesity induces other diseases such as hypertension, diabetes, etc. that greatly increase the morbidity and mortality from obesity.

One pundit has stated that obesity is second only to smoking as a preventable cause of death.

Etiology of Obesity

While "eating too much" may be a substantial cause for obesity, the disease is much more complex than that. Certainly when caloric intake exceeds caloric consumption over a prolonged period, fat will accumulate. However, there are poorly defined genetic, hormonal, and psychological factors that predispose some people to progressively worsening obesity even though their dietary intake may not be excessive. In addition, caloric consumption is highly leveraged with exercise, and many patients are unable to increase their metabolic rate by exercise because of pain, stress injuries, time or motivation. Psychological problems such as compulsive eating disorders are another cause of obesity. And finally, obesity might be drug induced such as from the use of steroids for arthritis, sedatives for anxiety, or the use of antidepressants. In men the excess fat tends to accumulate in the abdomen, while in women it accumulates in the hips, thighs and legs as well as the abdomen.

© Springer International Publishing Switzerland 2017
C.P. Larson Jr., R.A. Jaffe, *Practical Anesthetic Management*,
DOI 10.1007/978-3-319-42866-6_12

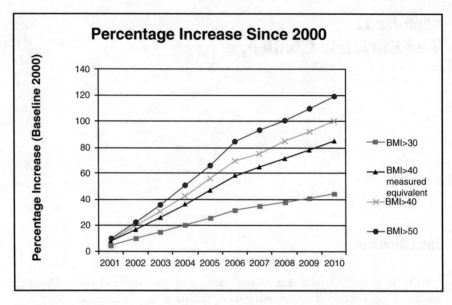

Fig. 12.1 Prevalence growth by severity of obesity (in percent over 1986 baseline). From Sturm, R., & Hattori, A. Morbid obesity rates continue to rise rapidly in the US. International Journal of Obesity (2013);37(6):889–891. Reprinted with permission from Nature Publishing Group

Classification of Obesity

Obesity is classified according to the body mass index (or BMI) expressed in weight in kilograms divided by height in meters squared (kg/m^2) or BMI = wt kg/ht m^2. The following are two examples of the calculation of BMI.

1. Woman 5 ft 4 in. tall weighing 126 lbs:

   126 lbs/2.2 kg/lb = 57 kg
   5 ft 4 in. or 64 in. × 2.54 cm/in. = 1.63 m × 2 = 3.25 m^2
   BMI = 57/3.25 = 18

2. Woman 5 ft 4 in. tall weighing 220 lbs:

   220 lbs/2.2 kg/lb = 100 kg
   5 ft 4 in. or 64 in. × 2.54 cm/in. = 1.63 m × 2 = 3.25 m^2
   BMI = 100/3.25 = 31

The BMI categories are shown on Table 12.1. As both the duration of the obesity and its severity (as measured by BMI) increase, obese patients become susceptible to a whole host of serious medical problems (co-morbid factors).

Table 12.1 Classification of obesity

BMI (kg/m^2)	Label
<18	Underweight
19–24	Normal weight
25–29	Overweight
30–39	Obese
>35	Morbidly obese of comorbid factors exist
>40	Morbidly obese
>50	Super obese

Medical consequences of obesity
A. Respiratory
1. Loss of lung volume (expiratory reserve volume) from abdominal distension
2. Hyperventilation to maintain adequate gas exchange
3. Respiratory insufficiency when lying supine or prone
4. Hypoventilation syndrome
5. Obstructive sleep apnea (OSA) from neck enlargement and excess fat deposits in the upper airway
B. Circulatory:
1. Systemic hypertension and subsequent left ventricular hypertrophy
2. Pulmonary hypertension
3. Dysrhythmias
4. Coronary artery disease
5. Thromboembolism causing sudden cardiac death or ischemic stroke
C. Gastrointestinal:
1. Gastroesophageal reflux disease (GERD)
2. Fatty liver syndrome
D. Metabolic:
1. Diabetes, type II
2. Metabolic syndrome

Obese patients may have any combination of these conditions, but the most common are hyperventilation and respiratory distress lying flat, hypertension, and diabetes, type II. While obstructive sleep apnea might be suspected by the obese patient and/or family, confirmation requires a polysomnogram or sleep study which most patients coming for bariatric surgery will not have had. However, it is reasonable to assume that those obese patients who present with a history of restless sleeping, pronounced snoring or observed episodes of apnea during sleep may have a component of obstructive sleep apnea. Some obese patients develop what has been termed "a metabolic syndrome", which is characterized by abdominal obesity, hypertension, increased fasting blood glucose levels, low levels of high density lipoprotein, increased serum triglycerides, and resistance to insulin. These patients are particularly prone to develop diabetes, and are at greater risk for death from their disease.

Medical Management of Obesity

Most obese patients initially try to control their weight gain by subscribing to or enrolling in one or more of a variety of commercial dietary plans. These efforts may be combined with utilization of "over the counter" medications that work as appetite suppressants, metabolic stimulants or as lipase inhibitors that block the absorption of some fats. Most patients are temporarily successful on a variety of dietary plans. However, numerous well-done comprehensive studies have shown that weight recidivism in morbidly obese patients on a program of organized diet and exercise ranges between 95 and 98 % in as little as 6 months. To make matters worse, the amount of weight regained nearly uniformly exceeds the amount of weight lost. Currently bariatric surgery has been established to be the only durable treatment for morbid obesity, and the continually improving safety profile for this treatment has increased the number of patients seeking and being referred for surgery.

However, before any consideration is given to bariatric surgery, obese patients must be given a sustained, comprehensive trial of medical therapy. This would include a structured dietary intake, a regular program of exercise to the extent that that is physically possible, cessation of smoking, control of blood sugar, and psychological or behavioral evaluation and support. In our system, patients must be on this life-style changing regime for a sustained period of time and demonstrate an ability to lose weight before they are considered candidates for bariatric surgery. The goal of our program is not to achieve dramatic weight loss, but to demonstrate that permanent behavioral modification is possible. Bariatric surgery without behavioral changes carries a significant risk of weight recidivism despite the anatomical alterations. In those circumstances, the patient has assumed all of the risks associated with surgery, and achieved none of the benefits. Additionally, if a patient regains all of the weight lost after surgery, the co-morbid disease processes return for good; meaning if a patient has remission of diabetes or hypertension due to weight loss from surgery and then regains weight resulting in return of disease, even future weight loss will not improve those conditions a second time. This is the reason that our program adamantly enforces preoperative demonstration of lifestyle changes.

Surgical Management of Obesity

The types of surgery performed fall into one of two categories in terms of effect. There are those operations that diminish gastric volume, so-called restrictive procedures, such as lap banding or sleeve gastrectomy, and those that combine gastric volume decrease with a component of malabsorbtion (Roux-en-y gastric bypass, duodenal switch). This type of diversion allows mixing of the smaller volumes of food, gastric juices and bile more distal in the alimentary route, which results in metabolically beneficial hormonal alterations. The length of small bowel bypassed is currently much shorter than was originally described in the 1960s, with identical benefits, thereby lessening the likelihood of long term nutritional disorders. Most bariatric surgery is performed laparoscopically, which results in less postoperative pain and shorter hospital stay (usually not more than 2 days).

Anesthetic Management

Preoperative Preparation

In addition to the standard preoperative evaluation (history, physical examination, laboratory studies) that accompanies any planned anesthetic, there are some special issues of importance in patients undergoing bariatric surgery.

Key issues for anesthesia
Preoperative
1. Prior history of difficult ventilation/intubation
2. History of hypertension and therapy
3. History of reflux and therapy
4. History of diabetes; use of hypoglycemic drugs
5. History of obstructive sleep apnea; sleep study
6. Complete airway examination
7. Standard bowel prep; fluid therapy preop
8. Subcutaneous heparin administration
Intraoperative
1. Positioning; thoracic elevation
2. Airway management
3. General vs. regional anesthesia
4. Drug choice and dosing
5. Monitoring
6. Fluid therapy
7. Extubation strategy
Postoperative
1. Pain control
2. Antiemetics

Since many bariatric patients have hypertension, and some have reflux, diabetes or obstructive sleep apnea, it is vital to characterize their condition(s) preoperatively. There is no evidence that bariatric patients are more susceptible to pulmonary aspiration than the non-obese. The American Heart Association (AHA) has recently published a science advisory on the cardiovascular evaluation and management of severely obese patients undergoing surgery [1]. This advisory is not directed specifically at patients undergoing bariatric surgery, but its recommendations certainly apply to bariatric surgery patients. In brief, if by clinical evaluation the cardiac risk is low, then the only special testing needed would be an electrocardiogram and chest x-ray. If the cardiovascular risk seems more substantial, then evaluation of functional capacity by stress testing is recommended. The value of more invasive testing such as angiography has not been established in this patient population, but may be appropriate in selected circumstances. If substantial respiratory impairment is suspected because of obesity, the AHA recommends obtaining a preoperative arterial blood gas analysis.

Although there is no consensus on this issue, both clinical studies and experience have shown that not all bariatric patients present as a difficult airway either in terms of ventilation or tracheal intubation. However, using the Intubation Difficulty Scale, two studies have shown that obese patients have higher scores than non-obese patients [2, 3]. The usual assessment of the airway including neck circumference and mobility, thyromental distance, Mallampati score, upper lip bite test, mouth opening, tongue size, presence of redundant jowls, etc. may suggest airway difficulty, but none are absolute indicators of ease or difficulty of ventilation or intubation. Most importantly, if a patient gives a history of difficult ventilation or intubation, it should be a red flag warning that alternate methods of airway management need to be available. The airway findings on physical examination should be documented on the preoperative anesthetic evaluation sheet.

Since patients undergoing laparoscopic bariatric surgery uniformly have a preoperative bowel prep, fluid therapy should be initiated while in the preoperative holding area. This is particularly important if the patient is hypertensive preoperatively. Administration of a liter or two of crystalloid solution before induction of anesthesia will lessen the incidence and severity of hypotension on induction of anesthesia. Finally, it is customary for surgeons to order for heparin to be administered subcutaneously just prior to surgery in expectation that it will decrease the likelihood of postoperative thromboembolism.

Intraoperative Management

Positioning

Positioning is a key issue in patients undergoing bariatric surgery, both for improving conditions for tracheal intubation, and ensuring the safety of patients during anesthesia and surgery. To facilitate endotracheal intubation, it has become standard practice in many centers to "ramp up" the patient by placing several bath blankets under the head and shoulders so that they are above the thorax. The major problem with "ramping" is that the bath blankets may have to be removed after tracheal intubation so that the patient can be properly positioned for surgery. Alternatively, we have found that a better positioning technique for tracheal intubation is to elevate the back of the operating table 30–40° and then drop the head so that the sternal notch is level with the ear canal. Once endotracheal intubation is accomplished, the optimum position for laparoscopic surgery requires the patient to be semi-standing, with moderate extension of the back. To ensure patient safety, the feet, legs and thighs are well padded, and then secured with tape at the thighs and just above the ankles.

Airway Management

As stated earlier, endotracheal intubation is often easily accomplished by direct laryngoscopy (Plan A, see Chap. 4). However, if the preoperative evaluation suggests that tracheal intubation may be difficult, or if on direct laryngoscopy the laryngeal opening is not visualized, then there are several alternative techniques for intubation that should be readily available. One is what is called Plan B [see Chap. 4] [4], which involves utilization of an intubating catheter (Frova or Cook catheter) or use of a video laryngoscope such as the GlideScope. If for whatever reason either or both of these should fail, the next option is Plan C. This involves inserting a standard LMA into the oropharynx, which is used as a conduit for a fiberoptic bronchoscope. A #6.0 uncuffed endotracheal tube is mounted on the bronchoscope, and the scope is then inserted into the larynx via the LMA. Then the 6.0 tube is advanced into the larynx using the scope as a guide. The scope is then removed, and ventilation of the lungs re-established via the 6.0 tube. When conditions are satisfactory, a medium size airway exchange catheter (e.g.: 4.8 OD, Hudson RCI, Teleflex Medical, Research Triangle Park, North Carolina, 27709) is inserted into the trachea via the 6.0 tube, the 6.0 tube is removed, and a 7.0 or 7.5 tracheal tube is inserted into the larynx using the airway exchange catheter as a conduit. With a little practice, Plan C can be accomplished in less than 5 min. It is well to remember that regardless of the intubation technique, smaller tubes are easier to insert than larger tubes. A 7.0 tube is suitable for most adults, and it would be rare to need a tube larger than 7.5.

Controlled ventilation is necessary throughout the operative period. Airway pressures required to maintain a normal Pa_{CO2} may be considerably higher than in other operative procedures because of the size of the endotracheal tube, and the upward pressure on the diaphragm caused by the pneumopertineum required to perform the operation.

General vs. Regional Anesthesia

When bariatric surgery was done as an open abdominal procedure, there was considerable merit to regional anesthesia, particularly for control of postoperative pain. However, with the laparoscopic approach, there is much less postoperative pain, and the main advantage of regional anesthesia is absent. Furthermore, because of the semi-sitting position for the surgery, general anesthesia would be necessary even if a regional block is used.

Drug Choice and Dosing

The first study that compared recovery times following desflurane or sevoflurane anesthesia found that they were consistently shorter with desflurane. However, several subsequent, better controlled studies have shown that recovery times are the same for desflurane and sevoflurane if the volatile anesthetic concentration is maintained at about MAC 1.4 or less (desflurane 8 %; sevoflurane 2.7 %). These or lower concentrations are quite adequate considering that other drugs such as opiates, propofol and midazolam are given at some point in the anesthetic care. Generally nitrous oxide is not used to avoid any possibility of bowel distension even though it has been demonstrated that surgeons are usually unable to discern if nitrous oxide is actually in use [4].

For most intravenous anesthetics and neuromuscular blocking drugs, it is advisable to select doses based on ideal body weight rather than total body weight. This is particularly true for propofol, opiates, rocuronium and vecuronium. Because bariatric patients have had a bowel prep and have a decreased circulating blood volume, rapid administration of propofol based on total body weight will often cause a profound hypotension. Likewise, because bariatric patients may have undiagnosed obstructive sleep apnea (OSA), intraoperative opiates should be used judiciously [5] and administered according to ideal body weight. Furthermore, substantial doses of opiates are not necessary for postoperative pain control, since in most patients the severity of pain is mild to moderate. Finally, neuromuscular blocking drugs should be administered cautiously based on ideal body weight and with monitoring of neuromuscular transmission. It is well to remember that once the operation is completed, closure of the laparoscopic ports generally takes only a few minutes.

Monitoring

Generally standard ASA monitoring is sufficient for patients undergoing bariatric surgery. For reliable, accurate blood pressure monitoring it is advisable to place the cuff on the forearm just below the elbow, and tape it in place so that it does not migrate down the forearm. This location works much better in most obese patients than putting the cuff on the arm, which is standard in non-obese patients. It is seldom necessary to place an arterial catheter for blood pressure monitoring. One caveat. Temperature monitoring should never be done by placing a probe in the esophagus, as it may end up in the stomach and be incorporated into the operative site. Any other location is fine.

Commonly the surgeons will request the placement of a special gastric tube with a distal balloon for localizing the operative site. In addition, once the operative procedure is completed, the tube is useful as a port for injecting indigo carmine dye solution 60–120 mL for determining the integrity of the suture lines in the stomach.

Fluid Therapy

Because of the bowel prep, early and vigorous fluid therapy is important to minimize intraoperative hypotension. Occasionally because of the obesity it can be difficult to find a suitable vein in the preoperative suite. If such should occur, we recommend consideration of an inhalation induction and placement of the intravenous catheter after the patient is anesthetized when it is easier to find a vein. It is rarely necessary to place a central venous catheter. Fluid therapy is best provided by a combination of crystalloid and colloid, the latter being albumin 5 %. Generally, the crystalloid volume rarely exceeds 3 L. It is rare to need to transfuse blood in patients undergoing bariatric surgery because of the operation.

Extubation Strategy

If a bariatric patient has proven to be difficult to ventilate during induction or the trachea is difficult to intubate, it is vital to have an exit strategy for managing the airway at the conclusion of the surgery. As with any patient emerging from anesthesia, it is necessary to assure full reversal of neuromuscular blockade; adequate, sustained spontaneous ventilation; a high concentration of oxygen in the exhaled gas; and elevation of the thorax relative to the abdomen to minimize loss of lung volume from abdominal compression on the diaphragm. If there is any concern regarding adequacy of ventilation after removal of the endotracheal tube, it is prudent to insert an airway exchange catheter (AEC) down the endotracheal tube before removing it. Then, if any ventilation issues should arise after extubation, it is easy to use the AEC as a conduit for reinsertion of an endotracheal tube. So long as the AEC does not touch the carina, the patient will tolerate the AEC without coughing and will be able to vocalize in a normal voice. Once it is determined that the patient is able to maintain a patent airway, the AEC can be removed.

Postoperative

The two main anesthetic issues in the early postoperative period are control of pain and prevention or treatment of nausea and vomiting. Usually at the conclusion of the operation, the surgeons infiltrate the skin overlying the operative ports with bupivacaine to lessen the pain from these sites. As a result, pain on emergence and in the early postoperative period is usually not severe. However, most patients will require some systemic analgesia for at least the first few hours postoperatively. For immediate pain control in the recovery room, meperidine 20 mg i/v every 10 min until relief is obtained is a good choice because of its rapid onset and minimal respiratory depression. Fentanyl in 50–100 μg boluses can also be used, but one must be cognizant of the possibility of sudden onset of apnea, and observe the patient carefully for 20–30 min after each dose. For sustained therapy once the pain is under control, it is best to consider use of patient controlled analgesia with dihydromorphone or morphine.

If a patient gives a history of nausea or vomiting after prior surgery, we administer antiemetics prophylactilly before leaving the operating room. Our usual routine, which has been very successful, is to administer odansatron 4 mg, metaclopromide 10 mg or droperidol 0.625 mg, and dexamethasone 10 mg about 30 min before the conclusion of the operation. Of course, this therapy must be continued by the surgeons after the patient has been discharged from the recovery room if it is to have a sustained effect.

Summary

Bariatric surgery is becoming increasingly used for the treatment of obesity that has failed medical management. As a result, more and more anesthesia providers will be called upon to provide expert anesthesia care for these patients. As with any surgical specialty, there are some unique features about which anesthesia providers should be aware if they are to provide competent care. This would include awareness that obesity may predispose to other medical conditions such as hypertension, diabetes, and obstructive sleep apnea. In addition, the standard bowel prep may result in severe hypotension on induction of anesthesia, and as well, the patient may present as a "difficult airway" in terms of ventilation of the lungs, intubation of the trachea or both. Appropriate measures to prevent or treat these events are part of the anesthetic preparation. Finally, selection of drugs and dosage based on ideal body weight rather than absolute weight is essential to minimize anesthetic overdose and prolonged postoperative recovery.

References

1. Poirier P, Alpert MA, Fleisher LA, Thompson PD, Sugerman HJ, Burke LE, Marceau P, Franklin BA; on behalf of the American Heart Association Obesity Committee of the Council on Nutrition, Physical Activity and Metabolism, Council on Cardiopulmonary Perioperative and Critical Care, Council on Cardiovascular Surgery and Anesthesia, Council on Cardiovascular Disease in the Young, Council on Cardiovascular Nursing, and Council on Clinical Cardiology. Cardiovascular evaluation and management of severely obese patients undergoing surgery: a science advisory from the American Heart Association. Circulation 2009;120:86–95.
2. Adnet F, Borron SW, Racine SX, Clemessy JL, Fournier JL, Plaisance P, Lapandry C. The intubation difficulty scale (IDS): proposal and evaluation of a new score characterizing the complexity of endotracheal intubation. Anesthesiology. 1997;87:1290–7.
3. Lavi R, Segal D, Ziser A. Predicting difficult airways using the intubation difficulty scale: a study comparing obese and non-obese patients. J Clin Anesth. 2009;21:264–7.
4. Brodsky JB, Lemmens HJ, Collins JS, Morton JM, Curet MJ, Brock-Utne JG. Nitrous oxide and laparoscopic bariatric surgery. Obes Surg. 2005;15:494–6.
5. Bolden N, Smith CE, Auckley D. Avoiding adverse outcomes in patients with obstructive sleep apnea (OSA): development and implementation of a perioperative OSA protocol. J Clin Anesth. 2009;21:286–93.

Chapter 13
Preventing Ischemic Optic Neuropathy during Posterior Spine Surgery

Unanticipated blindness is a devastating event for both patients and medical personnel when it is discovered following emergence from anesthesia and surgery. It is equally unsettling when it occurs in a colleague [1]. As a complication that is unexpected by all parties, it leads to introspection, analysis of the specific anesthetic and surgical procedure, and attempts to explain why it happened. Usually no clear explanation is forthcoming, and all involved are left with the unsettling question "Was something done wrong to cause this?" The patients and their families who must forever live with the consequences of unexpected blindness are adamant in their desire for a full understanding of why it occurred. When no good explanation for the cause of the blindness is given, these patients and families turn to the legal system for redress and compensation.

Postoperative blindness can occur following many types of surgical procedures, but the most frequent, and therefore problematic for anesthesia providers are those occurring following spine surgeries in the prone position. It may occur in patients who are otherwise "healthy". It also occurs in patients with known hypertension, diabetes and coronary artery disease without any concomitant adverse effects on other organs such as the heart, brain or kidneys. To understand this problem more fully, the American Society of Anesthesiologists (ASA) appointed a 12-member Task Force to "review and assess the current scientific literature; obtain expert consensus and public opinion; and develop a practice advisory". The practice advisory was published in 2006, and its *specific advisories* will be addressed in this chapter [2]. As well, in 1999 the Committee on Professional Liability of the ASA established an ASA Postoperative Visual Loss (POVL) Registry to collect cases of visual loss after non-ocular surgery. Data collection was from two sources: voluntary submission utilizing a previously developed data collection form; and from the ASA Closed Claims Project. In October 2006, Lee et al. published an analysis of 93 spine surgery cases with postoperative visual loss collected by the POVL Registry [3]. All the patients in the report had their operations over a 17 year period between 1987 and 2004. Both the Task Force and the Registry concluded that the cause of blindness in most of the patients investigated was due to ischemic optic neuropathy (ION) of unknown etiology, and developed several recommendations for consideration.

© Springer International Publishing Switzerland 2017
C.P. Larson Jr., R.A. Jaffe (eds.), *Practical Anesthetic Management*,
DOI 10.1007/978-3-319-42866-6_13

Incidence

The reported incidence of blindness following posterior spine surgery ranges from 0.013 to 0.36 % [4, 5], which suggests that the event is rare. However, this incidence is misleading for a variety of reasons. First, because until recently there was no required national reporting mechanism, not all cases were included in retrospective analyses of blindness after spine surgery. Second, there are many spine operations that are minor in terms of duration, extent of the surgical intervention, and blood loss (i.e.: diskectomy), which skew the denominator in the calculation of incidence, and greatly lower the true incidence for patients undergoing major posterior spine surgery such as spinal fusion with instrumentation. A better analysis of incidence would be to compare the number of cases of blindness seen with the number of cases of major posterior spinal surgery exceeding a specific time period, or with time as a continuous variable. Third, although we do not know the total number of major posterior spine surgeries performed between 1987 and 2004, the fact that the Registry was able to identify 83 cases of ION in that interval suggests that it is an ongoing problem of some magnitude. Finally, events labeled as "rare", regardless of severity, tend to receive less attention in busy medical practices because of the expectation that it will not happen. A recent study by Rubin et al. suggests that the incidence of ION decreased 2.7 fold from 1998 to 2012 [6]. The authors did not determine the cause(s) of this decrease. They did confirm earlier findings that aging, male sex, transfusion and obesity all increase the risk of ION. However, regardless of incidence, it is essential to do all that we can as anesthesia providers to minimize or prevent this event. To achieve this goal, certain issues need clarification and a plan of action developed that has the consensus of the anesthesia community.

Etiology

Blindness following posterior spine surgery may result from either central retinal artery occlusion (CRAO) or anterior or posterior ischemic optic neuropathy (AION/PION) [7] (Fig. 13.1). Since the clinical manifestations of AION and PION are similar, they are typically considered together as ischemic optic neuropathy (ION). ION is more common than CRAO. In the Registry study, 83 of 93 patients had ION; the remaining ten had CRAO. CRAO is usually unilateral whereas ION is almost always bilateral. It is generally believed that CRAO is caused by prolonged external pressure on the globe, while there is no established etiology for ION. Although blindness can occur at any age, it is most common in patients over age 40. Recovery of meaningful vision virtually never occurs with either injury.

Prevention of CRAO

Since CRAO is believed to be due to prolonged external pressure on the eyes, prevention is relatively straightforward. Placing the head in Mayfield 3-point fixation will eliminate any such pressure, and is a good choice if a prolonged operation is

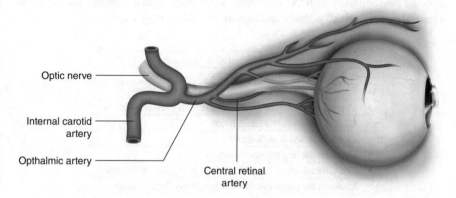

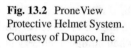

Fig. 13.1 Structural anatomy of the optic nerve and arteries

Fig. 13.2 ProneView
Protective Helmet System.
Courtesy of Dupaco, Inc

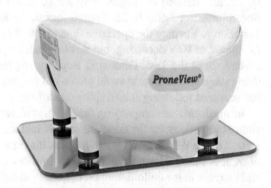

anticipated. Properly applied, the risks from using this head holder are inconsequential relative to the benefit. Alternatively, there are several available foam or gel-filled head holders with cutouts for the eyes, nose and chin. There is no evidence that one type is better than another, so long as the head is held in a neutral position, and all of the downward pressure is applied on the forehead and cheeks, and not on the eyes, nose or chin. The Task Force could not agree on whether eye checks should be performed by the anesthesia provider and how often. Certainly if technically feasible, it is probably prudent to do so periodically, recognizing that the examination itself may cause undesired head movement resulting in ocular pressure. Head movement for visualization of the eyes can be minimized by using a mirrored head holder (e.g. ProneView™) (Fig. 13.2).

Prevention of ION

Since the etiology of ION is unknown, it is impossible to provide any scientifically based recommendations for what to do to prevent it. The Task Force was not able to identify any predisposing medical conditions or any preoperative tests that might indicate susceptibility to ION. However, it did offer eight advisories for the management of "high risk" patients undergoing posterior spine surgery.

Task Force Advisories for "High Risk" patients
• Avoid direct pressure on the eyes
• Keep head in neutral position at or above heart level
• Consider insertion of arterial and central venous catheters
• Use colloid and crystalloid fluids
• Check hematocrit periodically
• Consider staging the operations
• Consider advising the patient of the possibility of blindness
• Evaluate the patient early postoperatively for blindness

They defined high-risk patients as those undergoing prolonged operations (not specifically defined but presumably >6 h), and/or those with substantial blood loss (the volume not defined). The conclusions of the Registry are similar to those of the Task Force. Keeping the operative time to less than 6 h would appear to decrease the likelihood of ION occurring, but this may not be possible when complex surgery is needed. Both the Task Force and Registry suggest that consideration be given to doing staged operations to avoid prolonged surgery at a single sitting. However, ION has occurred following staged spine operations, so this is clearly not the answer.

In an editorial accompanying the Rubin et al. report [6], Todd offered several possible explanations for the decrease in ION including use of the OSO/Jackson tables instead of the Wilson frame, shorter operating times, more minimally invasive operations, less blood administration, use of antifibrinolytic agents to lessen blood loss, and increase in the colloid fraction of nonblood fluids administered [7]. However, he omitted consideration of probably the most important reason for the decrease, namely the limitation in crystalloid fluid administration (see below).

Positioning

A variety of devices are used for positioning patients during posterior spine surgery, including the Wilson or Jackson frames or bolsters placed between the shoulders and hips. Once the patient is positioned, the Task Force recommends that there not be any external pressure on the eyes, that the head is in the neutral position, and that "high risk" patients are placed in a level or slight head up (reverse Trendelenburg) position. This is an important recommendation **for all prone patients**. The head up recommendation keeps the head in a less dependent position and decreases the likelihood of facial and upper airway edema, and probably ocular edema as well. It is very disturbing to family members to see pronounced facial edema postoperatively in their loved ones. To tell family members that the facial edema is a "normal" and unavoidable response to the surgery is somewhat disingenuous. The head up position may also lessen cerebral and venous pressures, which in turn may lessen venous congestion in the eyes.

Management of Blood Pressure

The Task Force recommended that blood pressure be monitored continuously (i.e.: arterial cannula) in "high risk" patients. However, it is often difficult to accurately and reliably predict surgical duration and/or blood loss in advance in patients undergoing spine surgery. Once the surgery is underway, it is challenging to place a percutaneous arterial catheter. Therefore, unless there is a contraindication to its use or impossible to perform, an arterial catheter should be strongly considered **in all patients undergoing spine surgery of any magnitude**, before they are positioned prone. Arterial cannulation has minimal risk and provides multiple benefits including accurate pressure readings during controlled hypotension. With arterial cannulation, one can avoid the limitation seen with cuff pressure monitoring, i.e.: unreliable cuff pressures if the arms are tuck at the sides of the patient and the surgeons lean against the cuff. An arterial cannula also gives easy access to blood for checking hematocrit, electrolytes and blood-gas values.

Some spine surgeons request controlled hypotension to lessen blood loss during posterior spine surgery. The Task Force did not believe that its use, per se, might result in blindness, and recommended that its use be determined on a case-by-case basis. If it is to be used, we have two recommendations not included in the Task Force report. First, the anesthesia provider and surgeon must settle in advance of the operation on a minimal acceptable pressure based on the patient's medical condition. There is no single value, such as 20 % below normal systolic pressure that is applicable to all patients, but in general a mean blood pressure greater than 75 mmHg would seem prudent. How the controlled hypotension is induced does not seem to have a measurable impact. Acceptable techniques include deepening the anesthetic level with volatile anesthetics and opiates, beta-adrenergic receptor blockade with drugs such as esmolol or metoprolol, alpha and beta-receptor blockade with labetalol, continuous vasodilator infusion, or some combination of these. Second, an issue not widely recognized or appreciated is the fact that if controlled hypotension is used, it rarely needs to be continued throughout the entire duration of the operation. Controlled hypotension is of greatest value during the early phases of the operation when the soft tissues and muscles are being dissected away from the spine. Once the instrumentation phase starts, bleeding is much less, and in most cases the blood pressure can be returned to more normal values.

Fluid Therapy

The Task Force made two recommendations regarding fluid therapy. First, colloid as well as crystalloid should be used when substantial (not defined) blood loss occurs. Second, monitoring of central venous pressure (CVP) should be considered in "high risk" patients. While the first recommendation is reasonable, it is not sufficient to prevent ION. The Registry report indicates that the average crystalloid volume administration in the 83 patients who developed ION was 9.7 ± 4.6 L. This means that at the extreme, some patients received more than 15 L of crystalloid fluid. These volumes are far in excess of what is needed and may be **the major contributor to ION**. In addition to causing facial and orbital edema, these volumes may create a **"compartment syndrome of the eyes"** or edema and ischemia of the optic nerves as they course through the optic canal.

We recommend that crystalloid fluid administration **not exceed 40 mL/kg regardless of the duration of the surgery**. If additional fluid is needed, which is usually the case, colloid such as hetastarch (not to exceed 20 mL/kg), albumin or blood should be administered [9]. Critics state that this recommendation is dogmatic and not supported by scientific data [10]. While true, it should also be acknowledged that there are no data to prove this recommendation wrong. The usual reasons for administering such large quantities of crystalloid solutions are either to maintain a reasonable urine output and/or to support the blood pressure. However, what is not widely appreciated is that urine volumes are frequently diminished in patients while in the prone position. Why this occurs or the mechanism(s) have not been determined, but may be related to the development of an abdominal compartment syndrome causing decreased renal perfusion. The common fear that patients in this type of surgery may develop serious renal insufficiency or renal failure if not given large volumes of crystalloid fluid has not been substantiated by research or clinical experience. Adherence to the crystalloid fluid volume recommended above will not result in patients developing serious renal complications if volume loss is adequately replaced with colloid or blood. Blood pressure support can be accomplished better with colloid since it remains intravascular for a longer interval. If after adequate fluid therapy blood pressure values are below the preset target, consideration should be given to utilizing a lighter plane of anesthesia and/or judicious administration of pressor agents.

Monitoring for Anemia

The Task Force recommends that hemoglobin or hematocrit values be measured periodically in "high risk" patients, but state that there are no specific values that would eliminate the occurrence of ION. ION can probably occur in the absence of anemia, but it is equally possible that the presence of anemia may increase the likelihood of a patient developing ION. In the Registry study, the lowest hematocrit was $26\pm5\%$, which means that some patients had hematocrit values less than 21%, which would decrease the oxygen carrying capacity of blood by about 50%. We recommend that periodic, intraoperative measurement of hemoglobin or hematocrit be performed **in every patient** undergoing spine surgery of any magnitude, not just those believed to be "high risk". This measurement is particularly important in those patients who have donated blood preoperatively. With only modest amounts of blood loss and fluid administration, the hematocrit may decrease to values well below the initial baseline. Determining the need for blood transfusion from estimated blood loss is too subjective and fraught with errors to be a reliable guide for transfusion. We recommend that hematocrit values be determined at least every 2 h (or more often if blood loss is vigorous), and transfusion initiated whenever the hematocrit reaches a nadir of 26%. While the Canadian Critical Care Trials Group found that a transfusion trigger of 7 g/dL (Hct 21 %) resulted in better outcomes in critically ill ICU patients than a trigger of 10 g/dL (Hct 30%), there is no evidence that these findings are relevant to patients undergoing spine surgery in the prone position [11].

Role of Research

While there are advocates for more research to determine the etiology and prevention of ION, exactly what research should be performed remains an enigma. Neither the Task Force nor the Registry offered any suggestions for studies that might shed light on the problem. Lee et al. [12] recently demonstrated that the optic nerve of the piglet is more susceptible to ischemia induced by euvolemic anemia alone or in combination with deliberate hypotension than is the corresponding cerebral cortex. While an interesting study, it offers no clues as to the etiology of ION in humans. We do not know if the same is true in humans, or what the role the prone position plays, and there is no ethical study that could be performed in humans that would answer these questions. Finally, if the mechanism is a compartment syndrome of the eyes from edema of the optic nerves and/or orbits, the Lee et al. findings may be irrelevant. At least for the foreseeable future, research studies are not going to resolve the problem of ION in posterior spine surgery.

The Future

The only reasonable course that offers any hope for decreasing or eliminating ION is to set some minimum guidelines for the care of these patients, and then over time compare outcomes with the historical precedence. The ten recommendations that we propose are:

Authors recommendations for preventing ION
1. Place arterial catheter preoperatively
2. Use head holder that protects eyes, nose, and chin
3. Keep head in neutral position at or above heart level
4. Establish with surgeon minimum acceptable blood pressure, with mean >75 mmHg
5. Limit controlled hypotension to dissection phase, not instrumentation phase
6. Limit crystalloid fluid to 5 mL/kg/h, not to exceed 40 mL/kg regardless of duration of surgery
7. Use hetastarch (up to 20 mL/kg), albumin or blood if additional fluids needed
8. Use colloids, lighter anesthesia and/or pressor drugs to maintain blood pressure
9. Check Hct regularly (every 2 h) and early in autologous donors
10. Transfuse at Hct < 26 %

While all of the recommendations in this list are important, the one that may have the most impact on preventing ION is the limitation in crystalloid fluid administration. Limiting crystalloid fluid administration to less than 40 mL/kg has several benefits. First, it greatly decreases the extracellular fluid volume in the head and eyes. Second, it lessens the total quantity of intravenous fluid administered, thereby lessening the onset and severity of anemia. Third, it lessens the likelihood of postoperative edema of the airway or congestion of the lungs. These ten recommendations are worthy of consideration, debate, possible modification, and implementation. Unless the anesthesia community develops some minimal recommendations that have the potential for influencing outcome, nothing will change and ION will continue to occur at the present rate. We desperately need to chart a new course in the care of these patients with the ultimate goal being to determine if minimum standards of care can be established. Trying these recommendations is the first step. Whether adherence to the recommendations provided will lessen or eliminate the occurrence of blindness in posterior spinal surgery remains to be seen, but it will serve to standardize care and make future analyses of this complication more meaningful. Resistance to this course of action because of medicolegal concerns can be readily addressed by indicating that this is a trial therapy, and that there is no evidence that the recommendations proposed will decrease the incidence or prevent the occurrence of ION,

References

1. Lehner AD. If my spine surgery went fine, why can't I see? Preoperative Visual Loss and Informed Consent. APFS Newsl. 2008;23:1–3.
2. American Society of Anesthesiologists Task Force on Perioperative Blindness. Practice advisory for perioperative visual loss associated with spine surgery: a report by the American Society of Anesthesiologists Task Force on Perioperative Blindness. Anesthesiology. 2006;104:1319–28.
3. Lee LA, Roth S, Posner KL, Cheney FW, Caplan RA, Newman NJ, Domino KB. The American Society of Anesthesiologists Postoperative Visual Loss Registry: analysis of 93 spine surgery cases with postoperative visual loss. Anesthesiology. 2006;105:652–9.
4. Patil CG, Lad EM, Lad SP, Ho C, Boakye M. Visual loss after spine surgery: a population-based study. Spine. 2008;13:1491–6.
5. Holy SE, Tsai JH, McAllister RK, Smith KH. Perioperative ischemic optic neuropathy. A case control analysis of 126,666 surgical procedures at a single institution. Anesthesiology. 2009;110:246–53.
6. Rubin DS, Parakati I, Lee LA, Moss HE, Joslin CE, Roth S. Perioperative visual loss in spine fusion surgery. Anesthesiology 2016;125:457–64.
7. Valerie B, Newman NJ. Ischemic optic neuropathies. N Engl J Med. 2015;372:2428–36.
8. Todd MM. Good news. But why is the incidence of postoperative ischemic optic neuropathy falling? Anesthesiology 2016;125:445–8.
9. Larson CP. Excessive crystalloid infusion may contribute to ischemic optic neuropathy. Anesthesiology. 2007;106:1249.
10. Warner MA. In reply. Anesthesiology. 2007;106:1251.
11. Hebert PC, Wells G, Blajchman MA, Marshall J, Martin C, Pagliarello G, Tweedale M, Schweitzer I, Yetisir E. A multicenter, randomized, controlled clinical trial of transfusion requirements in critical care. Transfusion Requirements in Critical Care Investigators, Canadian Critical Care Trials Group. N Engl J Med. 1999;340:409–17.
12. Lee LA, Deem S, Glenny RW, Townsend I, Moulding J, An D, Treggiari MM, Lam A. Effects of anemia and hypotension on porcine optic nerve blood flow and oxygen delivery. Anesthesiology. 2008;108:864–72.

Chapter 14
Continuous Spinal Anesthesia: A Lost Art

Spinal anesthesia continues to be an integral and essential component of anesthesia practice, but its use has for the most part evolved into a single injection routine. For a time, continuous spinal anesthesia was widely used, but fell into disrepute following case reports of permanent neurological injury after its use. The case scenarios involved injection of a local anesthetic, usually preservative-free lidocaine via a tiny catheter inserted into the subarachnoid space [1]. It was believed that the injected drug remained concentrated at the end of the catheter and that caused the neurological injury. As a result, continuous spinal anesthesia ceased to be taught in most anesthesia training programs, and became obsolete in most clinical practices. We believe that this is an unfortunate outcome for a very useful and safe anesthetic technique when used in an appropriate manner in properly-selected patients.

Patient Selection

Elderly patients, those above the age of 60 years are the ideal candidates for continuous spinal anesthesia when undergoing pelvic or lower extremity surgery. Hip or knee replacement surgery, lower extremity trauma or vascular surgery are excellent examples of where continuous spinal anesthesia can be the best choice for anesthetic management. The older the patient, the greater the benefits. What are the benefits? First, the spinal anesthetic will relieve the pain of the injury and/or surgery, and will provide excellent muscle relaxation for the surgeon. Second, the continuous technique will provide anesthesia for whatever duration of surgery is required. The anesthesia provider does not have to guess the likely duration of the operation as he/she would with a single-shot technique. Third, the total quantity of local anesthetic drug injected is much smaller than with a single-shot technique, because the amount of drug injected can be titrated to reach just above the analgesic level required for the operation. Fourth, because of the limited extent of the spinal level compared to a single-shot spinal, the likelihood of extensive sympathetic

© Springer International Publishing Switzerland 2017
C.P. Larson Jr., R.A. Jaffe, *Practical Anesthetic Management*,
DOI 10.1007/978-3-319-42866-6_14

blockade and hypotension or other complications from a higher level is much less. Finally, the amount of analgesic or sedative-hypnotic drugs that need to be administered during the operation is usually none or minimal. If the patient has been in pain, such as from a fractured hip, once the pain is relieved with a continuous spinal the patient will usually sleep throughout the operation.

Continuous Spinal Technique

The biggest drawback to doing a continuous spinal block is getting the patient into a position that permits performing the block. The ideal position is having the patient lie lateral with the operative side down or dependent with the legs and head flexed toward the abdomen. This may be a formidable task in patients who are in pain from a fracture or trauma, and may necessitate administration of a low dose of a short acting analgesic such as fentanyl or alfentanil to lessen the pain. Once the patient is in position, the remainder of the procedure is relatively easy.

The next step is identifying the ideal interspace, which is usually L_{2-3} or L_{3-4}. A standard adult epidural catheter set is opened for use. Once the anesthesia provider has been appropriately dressed and gloved and the back sterilely prepped and draped, local anesthesia is generously injected at the selected interspace. The anesthesia provider then inserts a 19 g epidural needle (e.g. Huber-tipped, Tuohy needle) into the interspace at a slightly cephalad angle. Because of bony spurs or ossification, the provider may have to redirect the needle several times or even go to another interspace. Once cerebrospinal fluid is obtained, it is important to inject a small amount of rapidly-acting local anesthetic before inserting the 20 g epidural catheter. The local anesthetic will prevent the patient from jumping or complaining should the catheter touch a nerve as it is being advanced. The catheter should only be advanced a few centimeters beyond the needle tip, and observed to drip CSF before removing the needle. If the catheter does not advance easily, it is advisable to insert the needle in another millimeter to insure that the bevel is fully in the subarachnoid space. Also, rotating the needle slightly to one side or the other may facilitate insertion of the catheter. Once the catheter is firmly secured and bandaged, the patient returned to the position required for the operation. Usually the dose of local anesthetic given to insert the catheter is sufficient to provide pain relief for the surgical positioning.

Choice of Local Anesthetic

Any local anesthetic can be used but our preference is for spinal lidocaine 5 % with 7.5 % dextrose because of its baricity, quick onset and reasonable duration. It is preservative-free, and once placed in the subarachnoid space it acts within 1–3 min to produce analgesia. One milliliter from the 2 mL vial, or 50 mg is diluted in a 2 mL syringe using either sterile saline or water (depending on desired baricity) from the epidural tray. Each mL then contains 25 mg of lidocaine. Usually 0.2 mL or 5 mg of drug is sufficient to relieve any discomfort from insertion of the catheter and positioning of the patient, and will provide analgesia within 1–2 min. Once the operation is underway, if the patient becomes restless or complains of pain, a 0.2 mL injection followed by ½ mL of sterile saline flush through the catheter will restore operating conditions within 2–3 min. For most operations the total dose of lidocaine will be less than 50 mg. Because the local anesthetic can be administered as needed, and the onset with lidocaine is very rapid, there is no advantage to adding epinephrine to the local anesthetic. A light, transport mask or nasal prongs is placed on the face to provide oxygen during the operation.

At the conclusion of the operation, the anesthesia provider can leave the catheter in place and allow the pain management service to use it for postoperative pain relief. If there is no such service, or it is advisable to remove the catheter because of planned postoperative anticoagulant therapy, we recommend injecting a mixture of preservative-free morphine (Duramorph™) 3–5 mg with fentanyl 100 mg via the catheter before its removal. For most elderly patients, the analgesia will last 18–24 h and this will be all of the analgesia they will need postoperatively.

Complications of Continuous Spinal Anesthesia

There are very few complications from the use of a continuous spinal technique in the elderly. Hypotension from sympathetic block seldom occurs because the dose of local anesthetic is small and the spinal level insufficient to cause any appreciable vasodilatation. Once an adequate block is established, the pain relief usually results in the patient sleeping with minimal or no sedative-hypnotic drugs. Nausea and/or vomiting, disorientation, confusion, restlessness or combativeness are rare from this anesthetic technique. The question always arises "Will the patient develop a post lumbar puncture headache because of the large needle inserted through the dura?" The answer to this is an unequivocal **NO**. The elderly have sufficient fibrosis and sclerosis of the supportive tissues surrounding the brain to prevent any shifting of the brain in the cranial vault despite the loss of CSF. Postoperative sitting or standing will not cause a spinal headache in this population. New onset backache rarely occurs even though a large needle is used.

Several investigators have questioned the use of lidocaine for spinal anesthesia because of reports of cauda equina syndrome, transient neurological symptoms, and radiculopathy following its use. The cases of cauda equina syndrome were associated with the use of very small catheters inserted into the subarachnoid space followed by injection of hyperbaric lidocaine 5 % [1]. With the technique described here, using a small dose of lidocaine per injection and a large catheter size, the chance for a patient developing a cauda equina syndrome postoperatively is virtually nil. The drug cannot concentrate in sufficient amount to cause the syndrome.

Transient neurological symptoms and radiculopathy (pain and dysesthesia in the buttocks and legs) have been reported following the injection of spinal lidocaine, usually as a single injection [2, 3]. These complications have been reported with other local anesthetics injected into the subarachnoid space, so the complications are not unique to lidocaine. In one study [3], the incidence of symptoms was higher with lidocaine than with prilocaine or bupivacaine, but the symptoms resolved in all lidocaine patients in both studies within 48 h. One author questions whether epinephrine may contribute to the neurological injuries associated with spinal lidocaine, and recommends that it probably should not be use [4].

Summary

Continuous spinal anesthesia is an ideal, safe, and highly effective anesthetic in selected elderly patients. Those 60 years and older undergoing hip or lower extremity surgery are excellent candidates for this technique. With this technique, hypotension from the anesthetic is rare, and the need for central nervous system analgesics and depressant drugs during the operation are limited or nil. Likewise, postoperative, positional headache from insertion of a 19 g needle through the dura will rarely occur. Unfortunately, the continuous technique is seldom taught in training programs because of the concern for temporary or permanent neurological injury following its use, especially when 5 % hyperbaric lidocaine is used to produce spinal anesthesia. However, it should be clear that there is no study documenting neurological injury following use of continuous spinal anesthesia using incremental 5 to 10 mg doses of diluted 5 % lidocaine injected through a standard epidural catheter. We have performed many such blocks without any evidence of postoperative neurologic injury.

References

1. Rigler M, Drasner K, Krejcie T, Yelich S, Scholnick F, DeFontes J, Bonher D. Cauda equina syndrome after continuous spinal anesthesia. Anesth Analg. 1991;72:275–81.
2. Martinez-Bourio R, Arzuaga M, Quintana JM, Aguilera L, Aguirre J, Saez-Eguilaz JL, Arizaga A. Incidence of transient neurologic symptoms after hyperbaric subarachnoid anesthesia with 5% lidocaine and 5% prilocaine. Anesthesiology. 1998;88:624–8.
3. Hampl KF, Heinzmann-Wiedmer S, Luginbuehl I, Harms C, Seeberger M, Schneider MC, Drasner K. Transient neurologic symptoms after spinal anesthesia: a lower incidence with prilocaine and bupivacaine than with lidocaine. Anesthesiology. 1998;88:629–33.
4. Drasner K. Lidocaine spinal anesthesia: a vanishing therapeutic index? Anesthesiology. 1997;87:469–72.

Chapter 15
Epidural Anesthesia: The Best Technique

Epidural anesthesia is an excellent anesthetic for many types of surgical procedures in the thorax, abdomen and lower extremities. When applicable, epidural anesthesia offers multiple advantages to patients as well as surgeons and anesthesia providers. Foremost among these is that as a continuous technique it can provide analgesia for operations of any length, and then be utilized in the postoperative period to provide analgesia for as long as deemed desirable. Depending upon the drugs selected for injection into the epidural space, and their volume and concentration, the anesthesia provider can provide analgesia, sensory or motor blockade or both over a wide area of the abdomen and extremities, or in a select area of the thorax, abdomen or legs. These choices are well described in the anesthesia literature. What are less well defined are the ideal technical aspects of performing an epidural.

Performing an Epidural

An epidural is best performed with the patient sitting because that position maximizes the flexion of the spine and optimizes the openings between the spinous processes. A second choice would be to have the patient lying laterally with the knees and head maximally flexed toward the abdomen. L_{2-3} or L_{3-4} are the ideal interspaces for performing the block, but it can also be performed at L_{4-5} or $L_5–S_1$, either in the midline or via a lateral approach. With the back prepped and draped, the anesthesia provider should inject a liberal dose of 1–2 % lidocaine at the chosen interspace, including the deeper tissues as well as the skin. If adequate local anesthesia is used, the remainder of the procedure should not be painful or even uncomfortable. A 19 g Huber-tipped, Tuohy, or similar needle is inserted in the midline, staying as close to the upper spinous process of the chosen interspace as possible, and directing the needle slightly cephalad. If bony tissue is encountered, move the needle more to the center of the interspace and continue to direct it slightly cephalad. If that is unsuccessful then move to the bottom of the interspace or move to another interspace.

© Springer International Publishing Switzerland 2017   125
C.P. Larson Jr., R.A. Jaffe, *Practical Anesthetic Management*,
DOI 10.1007/978-3-319-42866-6_15

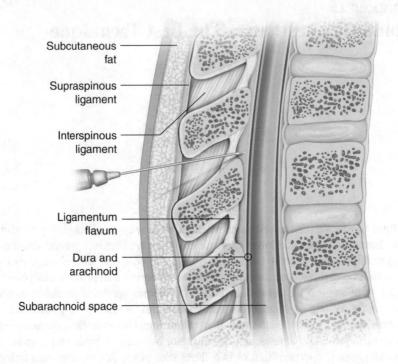

Fig. 15.1 Needle placement for an epidural injection

Once the needle is firmly fixed in the interspinous ligament, the needle is advanced slowly into the epidural space (Fig. 15.1). There are three ways to detect when the needle has reached the epidural space. The first is what is called "the hanging drop" technique. A drop of saline or water from the sterile tray is placed on the hub of the needle. The theory is that when the needle enters the epidural space, negative pressure in the space will suck the drop of fluid into the needle. Unfortunately it does not always work as expected, so most practitioners have abandon this technique. The second technique involves the principle of "loss of resistance". A 2 or 5 mL syringe, preferably glass or low friction plastic, is filled with sterile saline or water and a small air bubble is added. With each millimeter or less advancement of the needle, the syringe is balloted to detect if the air bubble compresses or if injection is suddenly possible, which occurs when the epidural space is entered. This is the most commonly used technique to identify the epidural space, but we believe that it is not entirely reliable. Since the ballotment is done after each advancement of the needle, it is entirely possible to inadvertently and unintentionally advance the needle beyond the epidural space, so that when testing, the needle is subdural or intrathecal, not epidural.

The third technique, and the one that we highly recommend, also uses the loss of resistance, but in what we believe is a more reliable method. Instead of putting an air bubble in the syringe, it should be filled only with saline. Instead of intermittently advancing and testing the syringe with pressure, a constant, firm pressure is maintained on the syringe plunger as the needle is **slowly** advanced. While the needle is in the interspinous ligaments, the plunger cannot be advanced. But as soon as the needle enters the epidural space, the plunger suddenly advances easily and the injection is easy. With continuous pressure on the non-compressible fluid as the needle is advanced, it is impossible to inadvertently go beyond the epidural space. At this point it is useful to empty the fluid in the syringe, fill it with 1 mm of air, and ballotte it after attaching it to the hub. If the needle tip is fully in the epidural space, the air will readily enter the epidural space. If the air does not enter easily, it is advisable to advance the needle very slightly until it does.

Inserting an epidural catheter can at times be difficult for reasons that are not evident to the operator. A few useful tips include rotating the needle slightly to one side or the other or advancing the needle very slightly while pushing on the catheter. Since the epidural space is only a potential space, it is always advisable to inject some fluid, either local anesthetic or saline into the epidural space **before** attempting to insert the catheter. When working in the lumbar region, we recommend that the operator inject at least 10 mL of fluid before inserting the catheter. For a thoracic epidural, we recommend 3–5 mL before inserting the catheter. If the epidural is being inserted for surgical or obstetrical anesthesia, the fluid in the syringe should be the local anesthetic to be used for the operation or delivery. The reason for this is that the biggest complaint that surgeons have about epidural anesthesia is the time that it takes from the start of anesthesia until the analgesia is adequate to permit the operation to commence. This time can be shortened if the initial dose of anesthetic is administered through the needle rather than waiting until the catheter is taped in place. The local anesthetic can be beginning to work while the catheter is being inserted and the epidural procedure completed. As well, inserting 5–10 mL fluid into the epidural space before inserting the catheter will lessen the chance for the local anesthetic to track along a narrow channel and producing a spotty block instead of covering the whole epidural space at the level of catheter insertion and beyond.

Summary

Epidural anesthesia is an excellent technique for many operative and obstetrical procedures. The continuous technique offers the special advantage of leaving the catheter in place for postoperative pain relief for as long as it is needed. The technique for inserting an epidural needle is best performed using loss of resistance with a small, fluid-filled syringe and maintaining continuous pressure as the needle is advanced. With this technique the operator cannot bypass the epidural space and inadvertently enter the subarachnoid space. Once in the epidural space, and a catheter is to be inserted, it is advisable to inject at least 10 mL of saline or local anesthetic before inserting the catheter in the lumbar region, or 5 mL in the thoracic region. This fluid injection converts the epidural space to a real space for the catheter, and prevents coiling of the catheter or spotty blocks from a channel injection if all of the fluid is administered through the catheter.

Chapter 16
An Incendiary Issue: Avoiding Operating Room Fires

Introduction

Oh no! Not again!! Not another operating room fire!!! How does this keep happening? Here we are, a very sophisticated, high technology country and we still can't seem to prevent fires in the operating room. Why is that? What are we doing wrong? While there has been a general awareness of operating room fires for many years, with many publications, especially in the journal Anesthesia and Analgesia, of fires occurring under various circumstances, operating room fires continue to occur. Because of this, the American Society of Anesthesiologists created a Task Force on Operating Room Fires, and their report appeared in Anesthesiology [1]. Included in the article is an Operating Room Fire Algorithm (Fig. 16.1), which, like most algorithms created by committee, is complex and difficult to remember in detail. To be useful in an emergency, it would need to be posted in a prominent location in each operating room, and this is what the ASA recommends. In addition to the ASA publication, the Anesthesia Patient Safety Foundation has prepared a short video on the prevention and management of operating room fires that is available for free by contacting the APSF (www.APSF.org). The APSF has also developed a simpler algorithm for fire prevention (Fig 16.2). The message from both sources is the same, and will be the essence of this chapter. Two case examples are provided to illustrate the types of issues that arise and result in an operating room fire.

Case One

The patient is an 84-year-old woman who was seen by her dermatologist because of a lesion on her nose. The dermatologist thought that the lesion was cancer so he referred her to a surgeon. Her history was significant for hypertension for which she

© Springer International Publishing Switzerland 2017
C.P. Larson Jr., R.A. Jaffe, *Practical Anesthetic Management*,
DOI 10.1007/978-3-319-42866-6_16

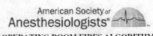

OPERATING ROOM FIRES ALGORITHM

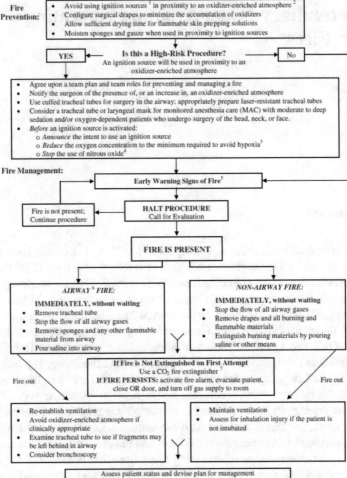

Fire Prevention:
- Avoid using ignition sources[1] in proximity to an oxidizer-enriched atmosphere[2]
- Configure surgical drapes to minimize the accumulation of oxidizers
- Allow sufficient drying time for flammable skin prepping solutions
- Moisten sponges and gauze when used in proximity to ignition sources

Is this a High-Risk Procedure?
An ignition source will be used in proximity to an oxidizer-enriched atmosphere

YES → No →

- Agree upon a team plan and team roles for preventing and managing a fire
- Notify the surgeon of the presence of, or an increase in, an oxidizer-enriched atmosphere
- Use cuffed tracheal tubes for surgery in the airway; appropriately prepare laser-resistant tracheal tubes
- Consider a tracheal tube or laryngeal mask for monitored anesthesia care (MAC) with moderate to deep sedation and/or oxygen-dependent patients who undergo surgery of the head, neck, or face.
- *Before* an ignition source is activated:
  - *Announce* the intent to use an ignition source
  - *Reduce* the oxygen concentration to the minimum required to avoid hypoxia[3]
  - *Stop* the use of nitrous oxide[4]

Fire Management:

Early Warning Signs of Fire[5]

Fire is not present; Continue procedure ← **HALT PROCEDURE** Call for Evaluation

FIRE IS PRESENT

AIRWAY[6] FIRE:

IMMEDIATELY, without waiting
- Remove tracheal tube
- Stop the flow of all airway gases
- Remove sponges and any other flammable material from airway
- Pour saline into airway

NON-AIRWAY FIRE:

IMMEDIATELY, without waiting
- Stop the flow of all airway gases
- Remove drapes and all burning and flammable materials
- Extinguish burning materials by pouring saline or other means

If Fire is Not Extinguished on First Attempt
Use a CO_2 fire extinguisher[7]
If FIRE PERSISTS: activate fire alarm, evacuate patient, close OR door, and turn off gas supply to room

Fire out

- Re-establish ventilation
- Avoid oxidizer-enriched atmosphere if clinically appropriate
- Examine tracheal tube to see if fragments may be left behind in airway
- Consider bronchoscopy

- Maintain ventilation
- Assess for inhalation injury if the patient is not intubated

Fire out

Assess patient status and devise plan for management

[1] Ignition sources include but are not limited to electrosurgery or electrocautery units and lasers.
[2] An oxidizer-enriched atmosphere occurs when there is any increase in oxygen concentration above room air level, and/or the presence of any concentration of nitrous oxide.
[3] After minimizing delivered oxygen, wait a period of time (*e.g.,* 1-3 min) before using an ignition source. For oxygen dependent patients, *reduce* supplemental oxygen delivery to the minimum required to avoid hypoxia. Monitor oxygenation with pulse oximetry, and if feasible, inspired, exhaled, and/or delivered oxygen concentration.
[4] After stopping the delivery of nitrous oxide, wait a period of time (*e.g.,* 1-3 min) before using an ignition source.
[5] Unexpected flash, flame, smoke or heat, unusual sounds (*e.g.,* a "pop," snap or "foomp") or odors, unexpected movement of drapes, discoloration of drapes or breathing circuit, unexpected patient movement or complaint.
[6] In this algorithm, airway fire refers to a fire in the airway or breathing circuit.
[7] A CO_2 fire extinguisher may be used on the patient if necessary.

Fig. 16.1 Operating room fire algorithm recommended by the American Society of Anesthesiologists (ASA). The ASA also recommends that this algorithm be posted in every operating room. From: Ref. [1]. Copyright © by the American Society of Anesthesiologists, reprinted with permission

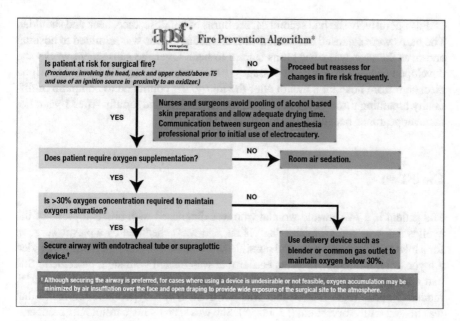

Fig. 16.2 Fire algorithm recommended by the Anesthesia Patient Safety Foundation (APSF). Reprinted with permission

took Norvasc 10 mg bid. In addition, she had a past history of congestive heart failure, although she was asymptomatic and her lungs were clear at this time. She had a history or coronary artery disease, and stents had been placed several years earlier. She had no history of chest pain or shortness of breath while walking or climbing a flight of stairs. She had a history of spinal stenosis and spondylolisthesis for which she took analgesics occasionally. Finally, she had a very recent right rotator cuff tear following a fall, for which she took analgesics (oxycodone) especially at bedtime.

After a complete workup, the surgeon admitted her to an outpatient facility for removal of the lesion on the nose. The plan was to excise it with electrocautery under monitored anesthesia care (MAC). The anesthesia provider applied all of the monitors and then attached a nasal cannula through which he delivered oxygen at 5 L/min. Just prior to the start of surgery, he administered midazolam 2 mg and fentanyl 100 mg to the patient. Shortly after the start of surgery, the patient complained of discomfort, so she was given both drugs in the same dose again. The lesion on the nose was excised with a cold knife and the bleeding controlled with the electrosurgical cautery. The tissue was sent to a pathologist who indicated that the margins were not clear, and recommended a wider excision. A second specimen was taken and the bleeding again controlled using the cautery. Shortly thereafter the surgeon noted flame under the drape. He removed the drape immediately and noted that the nasal cannula and oxygen delivery hose were burning. The anesthesia provider turned the oxygen off and removed the nasal cannula. In the process of removing the flaming drapes, the oxygen hose hit her right shoulder causing an additional burn.

Postoperatively she had second degree burns of her nose, face, neck and shoulder. The burns were cleansed and coated with Silvadene™. She was admitted to hospital and over the next week her burns started to heal. Over the subsequent weeks she developed stenosis of her nasal passages, which required surgical correction. Upon discharge from hospital a month after the injury, she continued to complain of difficulty breathing through her nose and pain in her face and mouth. After 1 year, her facial appearance became more tolerable for her.

Case Two

The patient is a 74-year-old woman who was diagnosed with bilateral ptosis of the eyelids that was compromising her vision, and was scheduled by a plastic surgeon for a bilateral blepharoplasty and possible brow elevation. Her past history included a myocardial infarction 12 years earlier that was treated with stent placement. She had a history of hypertension, which was treated with Losartan™, and Hyzaar™, moderate aortic regurgitation that was not treated, and hypercholesterolemia that was treated with atorvastatin (Lipitor™). She was seen by her cardiologist preoperatively and he concluded that she was only a mild risk for postoperative cardiothoracic complications as evidenced by her absence of any chest pain, shortness of breath or other symptoms, a recent negative stress echocardiogram, an unchanged EKG, and that she functioned normally at an oxygen saturation of 94 % breathing room air.

On the morning of surgery in the ambulatory surgery center, the surgeon announced that he would be using electrosurgical cautery to control bleeding, and that he needed the patient reasonably awake at the end of the blepharoplasty, so he could have the patient sit up and he could determine if any additional muscle resection was needed to correct the ptosis. The plan was to use local anesthesia on the eyelids and MAC with light sedation. The anesthesia provider insisted on using a mask instead of a nasal cannula for better oxygen provision. She trimmed the edges of the transport mask so they would not be in the surgical field. She turned the oxygen flow to 4–5 L/min. For sedation she gave the patient diphenhydramine 25 mg and hydromorphone 1 mg i/v.

The surgeon completed the operation on the right eyelid in about 45 min, and then started on the left eyelid. Shortly thereafter the surgeon noted a spark and then flames in the drape. He pulled off the drape and saw fire in the mask and oxygen tubing. The anesthesia provider shut off the oxygen flow and the scrub tech poured sterile water on the patient's face. A plastic surgeon was called to the OR and he diagnosed second and third degree burns of the face, nose eyelids and neck. Because of concern about an airway burn, the anesthesia provider administered a small dose of propofol (80 mg) and rocuronium (40 mg) and intubated the trachea. A pulmonologist came to the OR and did a bronchoscopy, which showed no injury to the larynx, trachea or bronchi. The wounds were coated with ointment and she was taken to the hospital ICU. Her trachea was extubated the next day and 4 days later she was transferred to a burn center. She remained at the burn center for several weeks, and had multiple surgical procedures to correct scar tissue formation. She remained blind in her left eye.

Hospital and Operating Room (OR) Fires

What do we know about hospital fires? There are more than 2000 hospital fires yearly and about 30 of them occur in the OR. However, the accuracy of these values is in question since there is no central reporting mechanism. Almost every hospital fire attracts local media attention because the public regards such an event as egregious. Almost immediately the legal profession becomes involved. Their thesis is that the care of the patient is under the exclusive control of the OR team; that accidental burns do not occur in the absence of negligence; that OR fires can be prevented; and that they result in severe disfigurement or death.

About 65 % of operating room fires involve a patient's face, neck or shoulders, as was the location in the two cases presented. Only about 35 % occur below the shoulders. The fire triad requires **a heat source, a fuel source, and an oxidizer**. There are multiple heat sources in an OR including the electrosurgical unit (Bovie™) which may be either unipolar or bipolar, hand held devices such as the harmonics scalpel, lasers, and fiberoptic lights. All of these devices are capable of providing an ignition or heat source. Although it is thought that the bipolar cautery is safer than the unipolar cautery because the current with the bipolar unit travels between the tips rather than from the application site to a distant grounding pad, there is no evidence to support this conclusion. Likewise there are many fuel sources in the OR including the patient's hair or beard, surgical drapes, patient gown or cap, and alcohol-based skin prep solutions. The most common oxidizers causing fire in the OR are oxygen and nitrous oxide. Ambient air with 21 % oxygen can support combustion but it rarely contributes to intraoperative fires.

Control of the oxidizer is a critical step in the prevention of OR fires. If oxygen delivery is essential, then strong consideration should be given to inserting an endotracheal tube, sealing the airway with the cuff, and if any work is to be done near the airway, placing wet gauze in the mouth and on the face. In most patients, continuous oxygen delivery is not essential, and it is rarely harmful to have the patient breath air and allow the oxygen saturation to gradually decrease to the 90–92 % range. Once at that level, and with the heat source inactivated, oxygen can then be given by mask, nasal cannula or endotracheal tube at high flows (6–8 L). At the same time controlled ventilation can be augmented or the patient instructed to breathe deeply until the oxygen saturation has returned to an acceptable level (97 % or more). Then the oxygen source can be turned off and after waiting a few minutes, the surgeon can resume using the heat source. The anesthesia provider can then resume administering air via the endotracheal tube, mask or nasal cannula. With this sequential technique, oxygen flow is rarely needed while the heat source is activated. There is no evidence that a nasal cannula is safer or riskier than a mask for oxygen delivery, so either is acceptable for use. For surgery about the face the surgeon usually prefers a nasal cannula because of its lower profile. There is also no evidence that continuous suctioning or vacuum extraction around the face or under the drapes offers any additional safety to the patient. During laser surgery of the vocal cords or tracheal dilatation, both of which are usually done under general anesthesia, the surgeon will often remove and reinsert the endotracheal tube multiple times. It is imperative that the anesthesia provider terminates oxygen delivery and administers air for several minutes before tube removal and laser therapy. Once the oxygen saturation reaches a near unacceptable level, the trachea can be reintubated, the cuff inflated with saline, and ventilation with oxygen continued. The cycle between administering oxygen, terminating oxygen and substituting air, and subsequent application of the heat source can be repeated multiple times either under general anesthesia or MAC. The critical thing is the maintenance of continuous communication between the surgeon and anesthesia provider so that both know when the oxygen is flowing and when the heat source is about to be applied. This communication eliminates any chance of use of a heat source while oxygen is being administered.

Case Analysis

With the information provided above, let's look at what went wrong in the two cases described in the beginning. Patient 1 had both chronic back pain and acute shoulder pain from the rotator cuff tear. As a result it is unlikely that she would be able to lie flat on an operating room table for any length of time without complaining or moving. A little sedation in combination with underlying pain may make her disinhibited and uncooperative. Enough sedation and analgesics to overcome this might make her likely to hypoventilate and readily develop hypoxemia, as well as become unresponsive to commands to breathe deeply. Knowing this before the surgery it might have been a better idea to insert an endotracheal tube, inflate the cuff, pack wet saline gauze or towels over the face, and administer air with the addition of oxygen ($FiO_2 < 0.3$) at as low a flow as needed to maintain adequate oxygen saturation either with controlled ventilation or spontaneous breathing. Alternatively, if it is decided to use MAC, then the oxygen must be turned off and air substituted whenever cautery is used. Even at low flow higher concentrations of oxygen would be dangerous.

The anesthesia provider for patient 2 was so preoccupied and concerned about the patient's history of a myocardial infarction 12 years earlier that she failed to recognize that the patient did not need an oxygen saturation of 100% to be safe. The preoperative studies clearly indicated that her heart status was both quite good and stable. The use of a specially constructed mask instead of nasal prongs did not offer any protection from a fire, and in fact may have made the transition from oxygen to an air environment slower because of the dead space of mask. The anesthesia provider should have utilized air as the inhaled gas and only administered oxygen when the saturation decreased below 92%, while having the surgeon stop utilizing the cautery. Both anesthesia providers were derelict in not establishing ongoing communication with the surgeon so as to correlate their activities such that the ignition source and oxidizer were not present simultaneously. This is something that should be clearly established during the "time out", and reviewed again prior to the start of laser therapy.

ASA Advisories

The ASA has developed a number of advisories to prevent a fire and to manage a fire if one should occur. A key advisory is the education of all operating room personnel to the possibility of a fire occurring by having at least annual lectures on fire safety and fire drills.

> **Education of Operating Room Personnel**
> Have periodic fire safety education
> Have periodic fire safety drills
> Know the location of fire extinguishers
> Post the fire algorithm in each operating room

Educators from the fire department usually give the lectures. These should be supplemented with teaching by local operating room personnel who are familiar with the location of the fire extinguishers in each operating room area, and the best exit route for patients and staff. There are a variety of fire extinguishers available, but most authorities favor the CO_2 type because CO_2 blankets a fire thus preventing it from restarting. In addition, CO_2 is cold so will not injure a patient, and the extinguishers are reliable and inexpensive and will not harm expensive electrical equipment in an operating room or radiology facility. Whenever possible, the fire extinguishers should be placed in the same location in operating rooms or hallways.

Prevention is the key to avoiding fires in operating rooms. A critical step in prevention is to question the possibility of a fire during the "time out" and to discuss among all operating room personnel what will be done to avoid such an event (Fig. 16.3). This is particularly important when doing a "laser time out" because of the special issues that arise when a laser is to be used. It should be affirmed that a laser tube is in place, that the cuffs of the tube are inflated with water, that there are moist towels surrounding the area where the laser is to be used, that the gas delivery to the lungs is air with minimal or no oxygen supplement; and that there will be continuous communication between the surgeon and anesthesia provider prior to and during laser use. The ASA believes that it is the **duty of every person in an operating room** to prevent a fire by speaking up if he/she believes that a fire is possible. Such concerns must be taken seriously and addressed appropriately before moving on. Where the risk of fire is high, each person in the operating room should be assigned a specific task should a fire occur. Such assignments will increase the efficiency in combating a fire should one occur.

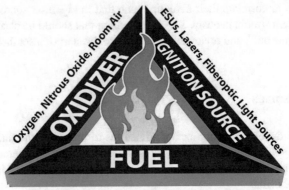

Alcohol-based Skin Preps, Surgical Drapes, Patient

Fig. 16.3 Prevention of fires. Question the fire risk during the surgical time out. If laser surgery is planned, review all of the special recommendations during the time out. Announce that every person in the OR is responsible for preventing a fire, and is to speak up should he/she have any concerns about what is to be done or what is going on. In high risk cases, assign each person in the OR a duty should a fire occur. www.fda.gov/preventingsurgicalfires

Once a fire does occur, its management may determine the severity of the injury to the patient and the staff. The first action by the anesthesia provider should be to turn off all of the airway gases. If the fire is in the airway, the endotracheal tube, LMA, nasal cannula or oral airway should be removed immediately.

What To Do If A Fire Occurs

Turn off all airway gases and stop surgery

Remove the burning materials from the patient; remove burning airway materials (LMA, ETT)

Douse the fire/flame on the patient with sterile water or wet towels

Activate the fire extinguisher; activate the fire alarm; call for help

Obtain immediate medical care for the patient

Quarantine all materials associated with the fire

Examine the ETT to make certain that it is intact

Debrief all parties ASAP to determine their recollections of the event

Notify the fire marshal and the regulatory agencies (state Dept. of Health, OSHA, etc.)

Review hospital policies regarding prevention/management of an OR fire

The surgeon should stop the operation and remove all of the drapes as rapidly as possible. If any part of the patient is burning, sterile saline or water should be poured on the fire or the area sprayed with the fire extinguisher. Once the fire is out, the site should be covered with wet, sterile towels. While this is going on, someone in the room should have activated the fire alarm and issued a call for help.

Once the immediate emergency is over, the next step is to provide medical care to the injured patient. If there is any suspicion that the fire involved the airway, an endotracheal tube should be inserted and a bronchoscopy done to assess any airway damage. Depending upon the type and location of the burn(s), the appropriate medical personnel should come to the operating room, evaluate the patient, and determine further treatment.

At this point the follow-up steps are very important to understand what exactly happened, why a fire occurred, and what should be done to prevent it from recurring. Often forgotten in the early follow-up phase is the need to quarantine all of the materials that were on or adjacent to the patient at the time of the fire. Whatever airway device was used should be inspected carefully to determine that all parts of it are intact. All of the personnel who were present when the fire occurred should meet with a facilitator and review what happened from their point of view. This is usually best done in a group setting so the participants can share what they remember and augment or clarify individual impressions of what happened. A detailed record should be kept of what is discussed. The hospital administrative personnel and legal counsel should notify the fire marshal promptly so the fire department can make its investigation. In many states it is also a requirement that the hospital notify state health agencies, Occupational Safety and Health (OSHA), and the Department of Health Services. Finally, the hospital medical and administrative staff should review their policies and practices to determine whether any new policies or changes in existing policies are needed as a result of the fire.

Summary

The vital issues in this chapter can be summarized in four sentences.

1. Prevention is the key; be aware that fires can and do occur in operating rooms.
2. Vigilance by **all operating room personnel** is essential.
3. Ongoing communication among all operating room personnel, but especially between the surgeon and the anesthesia provider is mandatory.
4. Utilization of air for patient ventilation is ideal; as much as possible avoid augmented oxygen or nitrous oxide in the inhaled gas mixture.

Reference

1. American Society of Anesthesiologists Task Force on Operating Room Fires. Practice advisory for the prevention and management of operating room fires. A report by the American Society of Anesthesiologists Task Force on Operating Room Fires. Anesthesiology. 2008;108:786–801.

Chapter 17
Tension Pneumothorax

Tension pneumothorax is a relatively rare event, and as a result when it does occur it is seldom diagnosed promptly and treated expeditiously. In hospitals, anesthesia providers are often called as first responders because the presenting problem may be acute respiratory or circulatory insufficiency. Thus, anesthesia providers must be aware of the condition, how to recognize it, and how to provide treatment.

Case One

A 52 year-old woman underwent a diagnostic right cervical node biopsy under general anesthesia at the patient's request. Anesthesia consisted of induction with propofol and maintenance with sevoflurane/nitrous oxide/oxygen breathing spontaneously via an LMA. At the conclusion of the 30-min procedure, the LMA was removed and the patient has a brief period of laryngospasm that was treated with bilateral pressure at the laryngospasm notch (see Chap. 5). By the time she reached the post-anesthesia care room, she was fully awake, conscious, responsive and breathing normally. She could take a deep breath without difficulty. About 30 min later, the patient stated to the recovery room nurse that she was having some difficulty breathing. The nurse listened to the patient's lungs but did not detect any abnormality. The patient's respiratory rate had increased from 10 to 18 breaths/min, but since her oxygen saturation was 97 % breathing room air, the nurse thought the problem might be anxiety, since the patient denied any pain. Ten minutes later the patient complained again of shortness of breath, so the nurse called the patient's surgeon. When he arrived, he noted that the oxygen saturation was 94 % breathing room air, the respiratory rate was 24/min, and that breath sounds seemed distant but similar bilaterally. He had the patient placed on mask oxygen at 2 L/min, ordered a chest x-ray and asked the anesthesia provider to come and evaluate the patient.

When the anesthesia provider arrived, he noted that the patient was having considerable respiratory distress, her oxygen saturation was 82 % on mask oxygen, and

© Springer International Publishing Switzerland 2017
139
C.P. Larson Jr., R.A. Jaffe, *Practical Anesthetic Management*,
DOI 10.1007/978-3-319-42866-6_17

her breath sounds were distant bilaterally. Over the next few minutes she appeared to lose consciousness and her blood pressure, which had been normal, was recorded as 52/37 mmHg and a pulse of 122 b/min. The anesthesia provider immediately took a 5 mL syringe, attached a 20 g 1½ needle, and inserted the needle into the right chest at the second intercostal space. The plunger of the syringe flew up and hit the ceiling putting a dent in the acoustic tile. The next blood pressure increased to 105/65 mmHg, the patient awakened, and with a deep breath the oxygen saturation increased to 93 %. A chest x-ray showed a pneumomediastinum and residual air in the right chest cavity outside the lung and a right chest tube was placed. A follow-up x-ray showed a normal left lung and full expansion of the right lung. The chest tube was removed the next day and the patient returned home.

Case Two

A 73-year-old man with a long-standing history of cigarette smoking underwent an emergency cholecystectomy under general anesthesia. The operation took about 90 min and the anesthetic was uneventful. In the post-anesthesia care unit the patient emerged from anesthesia and complained of incisional pain. He was given morphine 2 mg intravenously without any improvement. Over the next hour he was given morphine 8 mg in 2 mg incremental doses. After another hour the recovery room nurse called the anesthesia provider because the patient's blood pressure, which had been in the range of 165/78 mmHg had suddenly decreased to 85/52 mmHg, and his pulse had increased to 118 b/min. His oxygen saturation breathing mask oxygen at 4 L/min decreased from 94 to 77 %. The anesthesia provider grabbed an Ambu bag and mask and began positive pressure ventilation, which she noted was very difficult. At the same time she called for a chest x-ray. She listened quickly to the patient's chest and thought the breath sounds were diminished throughout the chest, but more so on the left side. The next blood pressure was 51/39 mmHg, so she took a 2 mL syringe with an 18 g 1½ needle and inserted into the left anterior chest at the third interspace. The plunger popped out of the syringe and air hissed from the barrel. The blood pressure increased and bag-mask ventilation became easier. A chest x-ray showed a partially expanded left lung, a fully expanded right lung and evidence of bullae in both lungs. A chest tube was placed in the left chest, and over the next several days the patient made an uneventful recovery.

Analysis

These two cases demonstrate a number of critical points in the diagnosis and management of a tension pneumothorax. One important point is that the presenting symptoms and/or signs may be protean in nature. In case one, the patient's initial complaint was shortness of breath or difficulty breathing, while in case two there were no presenting symptoms and the signs were primarily circulatory in nature. Whenever a patient develops symptoms or signs of respiratory or circulatory insufficiency, or both, the possible diagnosis of a tension pneumothorax should immediately come to mind. If the anesthesia provider does not think of this diagnosis, it is highly unlikely that she/he will manage the patient appropriately early in the patient's care.

What caused the tension pneumothorax in these two cases? In Case One the cause was aspiration of air through the wound site into the mediastinum and then into the right chest cavity. The transient partial airway obstruction from laryngo-spasm generated a higher negative intrapleural pressure, which may have enhanced the aspiration of air through the wound. In Case Two the cause was rupture of one or more bullae, which may have occurred spontaneously or was the result of positive pressure ventilation during the operation.

The first and most important step in diagnosis of a tension pneumothorax is having awareness that it might be the cause of a sudden, unexpected respiratory and/or circulatory insufficiency in a patient. Once suspected, the anesthesia provider should listen to the chest bilaterally, although it is often difficult to discern any appreciable differences in the intensity of breath sounds between the two lungs. One can also feel the neck to determine if there is any tracheal deviation, although this too is seldom useful. The anesthesia provider should call for an immediate chest x-ray to confirm the diagnosis. While waiting for the x-ray, several caveats must be observed. The first and most important is that the anesthesia provider should not leave the patient's bedside for any reason. A patient experiencing a tension pneumothorax can go from satisfactory vital signs to respiratory or circulatory failure very quickly. Second, if the patient has an oxygen saturation that is decreasing rapidly, attempts at positive pressure ventilation should be made. The question arises "Is the respiratory distress

Fig. 17.1 Needle decompression for tension pneumothorax. Insertion site of needle between second and fourth ribs medial to the anterior axillary line. The needle and attached syringe should be perpendicular to the skin surface upon insertion

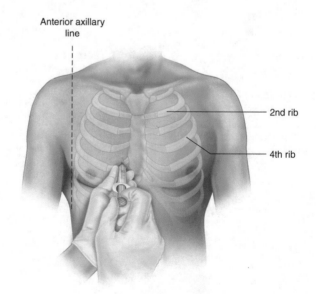

Anterior axillary line

2nd rib

4th rib

due to airway obstruction or a tension pneumothorax?" Attempting positive pressure ventilation may be both beneficial and a confirmatory test. Using a bag-mask or bag-LMA system, a high airway pressure will likely be necessary to achieve any appreciable increase in lung volume in either situation. If during the deflation cycle, the exhaled gas comes out of the nose/mouth quickly, as a jet of compressed air, it confirms that the gas in the lungs is under high pressure, which is diagnostic of a tension pneumothorax. If the exhaled gas comes out slowly, it is most likely airway obstruction. Third, the anesthesia provider must be prepared to insert a needle into the chest if severe circulatory failure occurs. The 20 or 18 g 1½ in. needle with an attached 2 or 5 mL syringe should be inserted in the second to fourth interspace medial to the anterior axillary line on the side where the pneumothorax is suspected (Fig. 17.1). If no air is detected on aspiration, then the same maneuver should be performed on the other side. Misdiagnosis of which side of the lung is compressed is of no matter since a chest tube can be placed on that side once the pneumothorax is decompressed. If a colleague is available, it would be helpful to have that person insert an arterial cannula in a radial artery for pressure and gas monitoring. Once the lung is expanded, the vital signs should return to more normal values very quickly unless the diagnostic period was excessively long or the patient has substantial underlying respiratory or cardiac disease unrelated to the pneumothorax.

Chapter 18
Tips on Blood-Gas Analysis

During cardiopulmonary resuscitation of a patient who sustained a cardiac arrest, the anesthesia provider asks a colleague to insert an arterial catheter and draw blood for blood-gas analysis. Shortly thereafter, the results are obtained, and the oxygen tension value is reported as 51 mmHg. The anesthesia provider says to the assistant "You must have drawn a venous sample." The assistant asserts with confidence that it was an arterial sample. He is right but how can he be so certain? The answer lies in the following analysis.

Consider the blood-gas values in a normal, healthy patient breathing room air, assuming a total partial pressure of one atmosphere or 760 mmHg (Table 18.1).

As arterial blood traverses the circulation into the venous system, the arterial oxygen tension decreases on average from 100 to 40 mmHg or a 60 mmHg reduction. At the same time the arterial carbon dioxide tension increases on average from 40 to 46 mmHg, a 6 mmHg increase. The partial pressure of water vapor, which is determined by temperature, (47 mmHg at 37 °C) remains unchanged since the temperature of the blood does not change in transit. The partial pressure of nitrogen remains the same between arterial and venous blood because the inspired concentration of nitrogen did not change and the tissue remains equilibrated with nitrogen at that atmospheric pressure, so no uptake occurs. The total pressure of all gases in arterial blood is 760 mmHg, but is only 706 mmHg in venous blood, a decrease of 54 mmHg.

Now consider the blood-gas values in the same patient under the same conditions with the only change being that the patient is breathing pure oxygen (Table 18.2).

First, notice that the carbon dioxide and water vapor pressures do not change as a result of breathing pure oxygen. What does change are the oxygen and nitrogen pressures. Since nitrogen is a very insoluble gas, it is not difficult to decrease its partial pressure to zero breathing pure oxygen through a non-rebreathing system for a period of time. If the total pressure remains at one atmosphere, the oxygen concentration must increase to 673 mmHg in arterial blood. However, in clinical practice it does not get to that value because of right-to-left shunts in the circulation (e.g.: Thebesian veins). A more realistic value would be in the range of 550 mmHg

© Springer International Publishing Switzerland 2017
C.P. Larson Jr., R.A. Jaffe, *Practical Anesthetic Management*,
DOI 10.1007/978-3-319-42866-6_18

Table 18.1 Partial pressure of gases in arterial and venous blood in a patient breathing room air at one atmosphere

Arterial blood		Venous blood	
PaO$_2$	100 mmHg	PvO$_2$	40 mmHg
PaCO$_2$	40 mmHg	PvCO$_2$	46 mmHg
P water vapor	47 mmHg	P water vapor	47 mmHg
P nitrogen	573 mmHg	P nitrogen	573 mmHg
Total pressure	760 mmHg	Total pressure	706 mmHg

Note the negative pressure in venous blood

Table 18.2 Partial pressure of gases in arterial and venous blood in a patient breathing 100 % oxygen at one atmosphere

Arterial blood		Venous blood	
PaO$_2$	673 mmHg	PvO$_2$	40 mmHg
PaCO$_2$	40 mmHg	PvCO$_2$	46 mmHg
P water vapor	47 mmHg	P water vapor	47 mmHg
P nitrogen	0 mmHg	P nitrogen	0 mmHg
Total pressure	760 mmHg	Total pressure	133 mmHg

Note the marked increase in negative pressure in venous blood when pure oxygen is breathed

for arterial PaO$_2$. While breathing pure oxygen will increase the solubility of oxygen in blood from 0.2 mL/100 mL plasma to 2 mL/100 mL plasma, it is not enough to increase the venous oxygen tension appreciably. The PvO$_2$ may increase slightly above 40 mmHg but it will not reach to 50 mmHg.

This analysis demonstrates two principles. First, the total pressure of all gases in the venous system is somewhat less than one atmosphere. That is, the venous blood is always under a slight negative total gas pressure. The difference in total gas pressure in the arterial and venous systems is markedly exaggerated when the patient breathes pure oxygen. The total gas pressure in the arterial system remains near 760 mmHg while in the venous system is in the range of 135–140 mmHg. This analysis answers the question why the assistant in the case problem cited in the introduction was correct when he asserted that it was an arterial sample. Even under the best of circumstance it would be difficult to obtain a venous oxygen tension of 51 mmHg, and certainly would not be possible in a patient who is undergoing cardiopulmonary resuscitation. It may be possible in some patients to increase the venous oxygen concentration somewhat by slapping the overlying skin vigorously before drawing blood from a vein (arterializing the local venous blood), but the oxygen change by this maneuver is modest and unpredictable. This analysis also demonstrates the importance of sealing a blood-gas sample as quickly as possible after it is drawn to prevent the sample from absorbing oxygen and nitrogen from air and distorting the results because the sample is under negative pressure.

Chapter 19
Preoxygenation

Several questions arise when considering the issue of preoxygenation. The first is "What is preoxygenation?" Preoxygenation is the removal of nitrogen from the body by oxygen. "Is preoxygenation the same as denitrogenation?" The answer is not exactly. With preoxygenation, oxygen is used as the sole agent, while denitrogenation is performed with oxygen combined with another gas in substantial concentration, usually nitrous oxide 50–60 %. "How much nitrogen has to be removed for the average patient to complete preoxygenation?" This value can be calculated reasonably accurately based on certain assumptions related to where the nitrogen is located.

The largest volume of nitrogen in the body is located in the lungs. Assuming a functional residual capacity (FRC) of 4 L and the lungs are filled with air that is 79 % nitrogen, the total volume of nitrogen would be 3160 mL. Nitrogen is dissolved in plasma in a volume of 1.28 mL/100 mL plasma at one atmosphere (760 mmHg) and 37 °C. If we assume a blood volume of 5 L and a hematocrit of 40, the volume of nitrogen in plasma would be 3000 mL × 1.28 mL/100 or 384 mL at a normal body temperature and atmospheric pressure. There is a small amount of air in the sinuses; middle ear and bowel, the exact amount of which would vary depending upon patient size and air swallowing, but the total would not exceed 20–30 mL. Most of the gas in the bowel is in the form of methane, carbon dioxide and hydrogen. So, the total quantity of retrievable nitrogen would less than 4 L in the average patient with 90 % of it being in the lungs.

'What must the anesthesia provider do to maximize efficiency during preoxygenation of a patient?' [1]. One essential action is to maximize the oxygen flow from the machine to the patient. There is no reason not to use a flow of 10 L/min, which is the maximal metered flow with most modern gas machines. The rationale for the high flow is not so much to replace the nitrogen in the lungs, which it will do, but more importantly to replace the nitrogen in the anesthetic circuit, whose volume is in the range of 7–8 L. Another important action is to maximize the mask fit to the patient's face to eliminate air entrainment. Often this is difficult to accomplish because of patient claustrophobia, edentulous state, facial hair or deformed facial structure just to name a few. A third action is to have the patient take very large breaths, which in

© Springer International Publishing Switzerland 2017
C.P. Larson Jr., R.A. Jaffe, *Practical Anesthetic Management*,
DOI 10.1007/978-3-319-42866-6_19

theory would hasten gas exchange in the lungs. However, big breaths will generate a higher trans-mask pressure (pressure difference between the inside and outside of the mask), which would promote air entrainment if there were any mask leak. Since mask leaks are common, it would more prudent to have the patient take normal volume breaths, which would keep the trans-mask pressure at 1 cmH$_2$O or less.

"How does the anesthesia provider know when the patient has achieved maximal preoxygenation?" Generally, most anesthesia providers settle for proceeding with anesthesia when the end-tidal oxygen concentration measures in the range of 80%. "Why not try to achieve 100% end tidal oxygen concentration?" Because it is not possible to attain 100% in the end-tidal gas for two reasons. First, there is carbon dioxide in the exhaled gas mixture. If the exhaled CO$_2$ is in the normal range of 35–40 mmHg, that would represent about 5% of the exhaled gas concentration at 760 mmHg. Second, while breathing oxygen the patient is consuming oxygen. If the inspired oxygen concentration is 21%, the average exhaled oxygen concentration is 15.5%, or a decrease of about 5.5% because of oxygen uptake. Consequently, under the very best circumstances, the highest end tidal oxygen concentration achievable during preoxygenation would be 89–90%. The anesthesia provider can speed up the preoxygenation process by augmenting patient-initiated ventilation, which increases tidal volume and maintains positive pressure under the mask.

"Assuming maximal preoxygenation, how much time does it provide before oxygen saturation in a patient decreases to 90%, a value below which most anesthesia providers would not like to go?" The answer is, it depends upon the circumstances. A normal healthy adult of average size breathing room air will desaturate to about 90% after about 2 min of apnea. Studies indicate that if the same patient is preoxygenated, oxygen saturation will remain above 90% for 8–10 min. In obese patients, the time is shortened to 2–3 min because of a higher cardiac output, decreased lung volume, and compression atelectasis from the weight of the chest and abdomen, causing right to left shunting of blood. Placing obese patients in a semi-sitting position during induction of anesthesia will increase the time frame before apnea induces desaturation. In patients with lung disease, the time from stopping preoxygenation to desaturation may be a minute or less.

Reference

1. Edmark L, Kostova-Aherdan K, Enlund M, Hedenstierna G. Optimal oxygen concentration during induction of general anesthesia. Anesthesiology. 2003;98:28–33.

Chapter 20
Diffusion Hypoxia

Diffusion hypoxia is a poorly understood event in clinical anesthesia. It occurs in only one circumstance, which is only when a patient simultaneously breathes two relatively insoluble gases, both in high concentration [1]. For example, supposing a patient is breathing nitrous oxide 60 % as part of a standard anesthetic technique, and at the end of the anesthetic is immediately allowed to breathe room air, which contains 79 % nitrogen. As the patient inhales, the nitrogen enters the lungs, but because of its insolubility does not enter the pulmonary blood stream in any appreciable amount. Simultaneously nitrous oxide, which is also insoluble but less so than nitrogen, leaves the pulmonary blood, enters the alveoli and is exhaled. If nitrous oxide and nitrogen had the same solubility coefficient, there would be an even exchange of molecules across alveoli and diffusion hypoxia would not occur. However, because nitrogen is less soluble than nitrous oxide, the molecular exchange of gases in the lung is not even. Nitrogen tends to stay in the alveoli and nitrous oxide continues to diffuse from blood stream into alveoli. As a result, the two insoluble gases concentrate in the lung thereby decreasing the concentration of oxygen resulting in transient diffusion hypoxia (Fig. 20.1) [1]. The same event could occur if one of the gases is a high concentration of helium. To avoid this problem, the anesthesia provider should always administer a high concentration of oxygen for a few minutes before transitioning from nitrous oxide (or helium) to room air.

© Springer International Publishing Switzerland 2017
C.P. Larson Jr., R.A. Jaffe, *Practical Anesthetic Management*,
DOI 10.1007/978-3-319-42866-6_20

Fig. 20.1 At time zero, the inspired gas was changed from 21 % oxygen/79 % nitrous oxide to 21 % oxygen/79 % nitrogen. Arterial oxygen subsequently fell in association with the outpouring of nitrous oxide (data from Ref. [1])

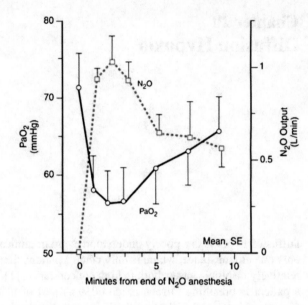

Reference

1. Sheffer L, Steffenson JL, Birch AA. Nitrous oxide-induced diffusion hypoxia in patients breathing spontaneously. Anesthesiology. 1972;37:436–9.

Index

© Springer International Publishing Switzerland 2017   149
C.P. Larson Jr., R.A. Jaffe, *Practical Anesthetic Management*,
DOI 10.1007/978-3-319-42866-6

Printed in the United States
By Bookmasters